ACCIDENTAL HEALTH

A MEMOIR OF
A UNIQUE JOURNEY
TO TRUE HEALTH

DEE MCGUIRE

For Gretchen, Kenny, and Chris
My love and joy

CONTENTS

Chapter One

TODAY

I waved to the neighbors and jogged up the three steps to our house. As I slipped my key into the lock I could feel heat radiating from the metal door that received direct sunlight most of the day. That warmth reminded me that I was home, and could slow the hectic pace that had defined the previous twelve hours. After a full day of work and several errands, I was looking forward to a quiet evening with the kids.

My son Kenny was home from college and my daughter Gretchen had taken the day off work to spend with him. My youngest, Chris, a high school student, had been in school all day, followed immediately by karate class. Chris juggled several large bags of karate gear as he came up the steps behind me. He sidestepped past me at the door and dropped his bags inside, loosening the long purple belt knotted low around his waist as he rushed to the back of the house to find Gretchen and Kenny. I knew it was torture for him to be gone all day while his siblings were home.

I pushed the bags aside with my foot, then tossed my keys onto a small wooden table next to a scattered stack of mail just inside the door. As I flipped through flyers for lawn service and window replacement, Gret bounded toward me followed by her brothers. "Hey Mom, do you want to play tennis?" she asked. "We can all go." The boys, several inches taller than Gret, flanked her like bodyguards. They smiled and nodded.

"It's okay, Mom," Chris said. "I can do my homework tomorrow during study hall." He seemed just as eager as his siblings, who had probably been lounging around the house all day.

What about dinner? I wondered, glancing at my watch.

"We can pick up burgers after," Gret said, reading my mind.

My tired body sagged for just an instant before a wide grin spread across my face. I loved playing tennis with the kids, and it was a gorgeous seventy degrees outside.

"Okay!" I said. "Let me change."

I was wearing slacks and a blouse that I put on for work at six o'clock in the morning, and low heels I'd regretted wearing when I rushed through a massive pet supply warehouse looking for dog food while Chris was in karate class.

We gathered our rackets and tried to find tennis balls that would bounce, a task made much more difficult as Honey, our seventy-five-pound Plott hound, and Bentley, a sixteen-pound miniature schnauzer, snatched the balls and ran through the house with them. Their little game was only enhanced when Chris ran after them yelling, "OFF! OFF!" with his purple belt trailing behind him.

It was dark by the time we left the house.

"Let's walk," Gret said.

She was a conservationist before conservationists were cool and didn't think it was necessary to start up the car for a two-block ride to the courts. The boys grumbled, arguing that if the courts were full we would have to walk a mile to the next ones with lights. I was concerned about getting to bed at a reasonable hour and had a nagging suspicion that I needed to get creative with the food left in the refrigerator to put together lunches for the next day.

"Let's drive," I said. "It'll give us more time to play."

We weren't good. At all. None of us. We were happy when we kept the ball inside the fence and avoided running into each other.

When we actually returned a ball over the net, we were ecstatic.

After an hour of extreme cardio, mostly from our heroic efforts to prevent our tennis balls from interrupting the game next to us, we began swatting bugs. They seemed especially big and fearless, and we lost interest in tennis as they began to swarm around our heads. Because of our shared gene for bug fear, and were all happy to pile in the car when someone mentioned dinner.

I drove a couple of miles to our favorite hamburger restaurant and we entered the queue to order. We studied the menu board behind the row of cashiers while our mouths watered from the smell of grilled beef and fresh brownies. Televisions blasting commentary for several sporting events combined with loud conversation and the excited screams of children playing arcade games created a very festive atmosphere. Once the kids and I determined that we wanted the exact the same food that we ordered every single time, we turned to each other bunched together in line.

"Hey, how do you like those tennis shoes?" Gret asked, bumping my foot with hers.

I wiggled my toes inside my sneakers. For years, because of debilitating back pain I could wear only a single pair of highly specialized shoes, full of inserts and cushions. The new ones I wore were just regular off-the-shelf athletic shoes.

"They're great!" I said. "I can't believe I'm wearing them."

"*I* can't believe you're playing tennis!" Kenny said, laughing and leaning into me with his shoulder.

We ordered, then moved to a table to wait for our food.

Chris explained to Gret and Kenny that my health was no longer a factor in our plans. As he described our day-long hikes and intense gym workouts, I thought about how much had changed. Three years earlier I could hardly function and truly thought I would've been dead by now. Even after more than twenty surgeries, countless invasive procedures, and a dozen diagnoses for chronic conditions, I'd continued to develop new symptoms that affected every system in my body and every aspect of my life. I couldn't sit, stand, walk, or sleep normally because of joint pain. My skin was pale, cracked, and infected, and I was exhausted all the time. I couldn't maintain a normal body temperature and couldn't focus long enough to address the simplest responsibilities at work and home. I was despondent and disengaged. But now, three years after I thought all was lost, I was healthier than I had ever been in my life.

This dramatic turnaround was not due to a scientific breakthrough or a new test result. The answer was shockingly simple and had been there all along. I found it by accident.

Now I took nothing for granted. I was absolutely thrilled to be able to perform the most routine tasks, and overjoyed to spend time with the kids. I was energetic and optimistic for the first time in years.

Gret and Ken each gave me a big hug, which brought tears to my eyes. They smiled warmly at Chris and told him how lucky he was. Then we began planning our next weekend together.

Chapter Two

EARLY DAYS

My brothers and I were very active kids. We grew up in Tennessee, where there was no reason to be indoors unless you were sick or sleeping. Video games, home computers, and movie rentals did not yet exist, and our television received only four channels if the antenna was oriented just right, so there was not much to keep us inside.

As young children we spent most of our time in a heavily wooded area we called "bouncy land," because the vegetation was so dense we walked on bouncy brush and rarely stepped on solid ground. We swung on vines over creeks and waded in the cool water, turning over rocks in search of crawdads and salamanders. We cleared paths with small hatchets and cut forts into the brushwood where we stored our prized possessions, such as snake skins, pointy sticks, lucky rabbit's feet, empty snail shells, and shiny pebbles. We were expected at home for lunch and dinner, but often picked apples, cherries, or plums from farms nearby for a snack between meals. I was always disappointed when the sun set and it was time to go inside.

After my third-grade year my family moved from our small, quiet neighborhood to a large apartment complex in a heavily populated area near the interstate. We left our tranquil bouncy land behind but quickly discovered the benefits of living in the middle of a huge group of very active kids. There was always something to do and someone to play with. We simply walked outside at any time of the day or night and quickly assessed the clusters of activity to determine which one we wanted to join. Kids constantly raced through the complex on bicycles and skateboards, no doubt to the terror of adults trying to navigate a car through a mob of children. We challenged each others' jump rope and pogo stick records and developed new skills, such as juggling and stilt walking. I even learned to ride a unicycle.

Our family moved away from the apartments and into a single-family home when I entered junior high school. The constant chaotic activity at home was gone, but I naturally transitioned to organized clubs and sports at school. I joined student government, ran track, and played softball and volleyball. I began working when I was fourteen and discovered how good I felt when I was busy and productive.

My older brother and I were still drawn to the rugged outdoors and regularly tossed our sleeping bags and pup tent into our shared Volkswagen Beetle and drove a couple of hours to Fall Creek Falls State Park, where we could hike and swim at the base of the waterfalls. When we weren't able to get a few days away from home, we raced motorcycles off-road or fished and swam in the coves of one of the nearby lakes.

By the time I entered college I enjoyed pushing myself and constantly looked for new challenges. I played powder puff football, rugby, was a goalie for the women's soccer team, and held three part-time jobs to help pay for school. For fun I trained with our marine corps ROTC cadets preparing for Officer Candidates School, and rappelled off the molecular biology building with the army cadets. I felt content when I was physically exhausted at the end of the day, restless and unfocused when not in motion.

Since childhood I'd wanted to be a doctor. I couldn't imagine anything more satisfying than working with all kinds of people to help solve all kinds of health problems. I was particularly interested in emergency medicine, because it sounded demanding and exciting. I imagined facing unique situations every day that required split-second decision making to save lives.

Volunteering at the university hospital emergency department taught me that much of the time was spent treating ear infections and stomach viruses, but there were plenty of thrilling cases requiring imagination and quick action from the physicians. In just one evening I saw doctors treating one man for a heart attack and another for a drug overdose while victims of a multicar accident were rushed in. Just minutes later a construction worker whose arm had been twisted off by a cement mixer was wheeled in at the same time as a hunter who was shot through the leg with an arrow. I was hooked.

In college I took all the prerequisite classes for medical school, with a major in biology. During junior year I started dating Phil, a funny and driven honor student with a double major in political science and sociology. He was studious and disciplined, a nice balance to my spontaneous nature. The single class we took together was Deviant Behavior and Social Control, a course in Phil's major and an elective for me. Each day after class Phil would review all of his notes since the beginning of the semester and complete any assigned reading, the same habit he practiced for all of his classes. When exams rolled around he was completely prepared and had no need for additional studying. This worked great for me because I was able to borrow his textbook, since I hadn't purchased one for myself.

By senior year Phil and I were engaged and planning our life together. I took medical school entrance exams but decided to take some time before applying to medical school. I wanted to graduate, get married, and relocate to northern Virginia, where Phil had a job and family before committing to an intense graduate program, possibly in another state.

Over time, the appeal of becoming a doctor was weakened by a more practical consideration. I had always pictured myself with a house full of active kids, and I didn't see how I could be the involved mom I wanted to be and a committed doctor. I volunteered as an emergency medical technician at a busy fire department when it fit my schedule, happy to find a flexible opportunity to stay engaged in the medical field.

I went to work in a research lab and took graduate classes, ultimately earning a master's degree in environmental biology. I found the research fascinating, and enjoyed the predictable work schedule, which allowed me to pick up part-time jobs to help pay student loans. Phil and I joined a co-ed softball team, and I played indoor soccer.

With the guidance of a neighbor and instructions from a *Time Life* book series on home improvement, I finished the basement of our town house, every step from framing walls and building out a ventilation system to tacking up wooden molding and recessing overhead lights. The project took over a year to finish because of my busy schedule, but I enjoyed every demanding minute of it. When it was finished, I was very proud of the new living space but missed my time with a tape measure in hand and drywall dust in my hair.

Chapter Three

THE BEGINNING

In my late twenties I became pregnant with our first child, and began to experience severe pain in my lower back. I'd suffered from back pain since high school, so I was used to sore or tight muscles when I bent or stood up from a chair, especially after running on a hard surface or sitting on a hard seat. But I was surprised by the new sharp and constant pain that escalated in intensity throughout my pregnancy.

I'd never really wondered why my back hurt before. I just assumed it was the result of demanding physical activity. Many of my older family members had a "bad back," so my back pain did not seem unusual. Plus, back pain during pregnancy was very common according to my obstetrician, caused by weight gain and changes to the curvature of the spine. The familiar image of a pregnant woman with one hand on a round belly and the other on the small of her back further validated for me that I was not experiencing anything unusual.

I was excited about becoming a mother, but had no idea until Gretchen was born that I could feel such unconditional love for a demanding little person I didn't even really know. She was perfect. I wanted nothing more than to keep her safe and show her everything. She became a curious and determined toddler, laser focused on pushing wooden puzzle pieces into the right slots and stacking books on her shelf until done to her satisfaction. She responded to any offer for help with a firm push away and an adamant, "*I* do it!"

Fortunately, my back pain returned to its prepregnancy level soon after Gretchen was born, though I was a little more sensitive. I was able to play with Gret on the floor and carry her on my hip with no problem as long as I was careful. Any sudden twist caused muscle spasms, and when I sat down too hard I felt sharp pain. I also found I was most comfortable sleeping on my side with my knees slightly bent. If I woke up with my legs straight, the muscles in my lower back would cramp violently when I moved them.

My second pregnancy, with Kenny two years later, was similar to the first. I did notice a slight but consistent burning and tightness in my lower back that never really went away after he was born, but there weren't any significant changes to my earlier condition.

Little Kenny had the determination of his big sister, but he was much more physical. He was not only walking by his first birthday but also running. Phil and I quickly realized the futility of baby gates, since Kenny could hitch his leg across the top and flop over like a sack of potatoes. He bounced up on the other side and immediately raced off with a big smile of freedom.

My pregnancy with Chris three years later was different. In the *first* trimester I was suffering with back pain at a level I had only experienced during the last few weeks of my previous two pregnancies. I couldn't sit or sleep for more than a few minutes at a time, and was unable to carry two- and four-year-old Gret and Kenny, bend to ties shoes, lean over for a good-night kiss, give baths, or pick up toys. I was often not able to drive, and was forced to reduce my work hours due to my inability to focus on anything other than my pain.

My obstetrician was so concerned by my condition (or so tired of hearing about it) he induced labor two weeks before I was due to deliver. I was relieved, and very anxious to return to my active lifestyle. Phil had taken time off work to be home as much as possible during my pregnancy, but would quickly return to his busy job as federal agent with a heavy travel schedule. I needed to be able to take care of three little kids on my own.

I soon realized that my recovery from this pregnancy was going to be different from the previous two. As my body healed, my back was not getting better. A consistent burning ache in my lower back became a stabbing pain with the slightest twist or bend of my spine. Sudden movement from a sneeze or a bump from one of the kids would cause a pain so intense my knees would buckle. I struggled to remain optimistic as time passed and my back did not improve. I desperately wanted to snuggle and play with the kids, but was driven to caution by an overwhelming fear of pain.

Chris was a calm and quiet baby, and was thrilled with the entertainment provided by his older sister and brother. Gret, happy to rediscover favorite board books from her early childhood, told stories to Chris for hours. He loved the variety of voices she used for different characters, more entranced by her expressions and gestures that the actual book. Kenny provided busts of unexpected delight, popping into Chris's face with a quick goofy sound or silly face, then zooming away again, leaving Chris in fits of laughter.

My heightened sensitivity to movement required new approaches to some routine activities, including Chris's bedtime. Bending to place him in his crib or lift him out caused my back to spasm and to shoot pain through my body that was so intense I couldn't breathe. To pick him up I would lower the rail, squat straight down like a baseball catcher, pull him by his clothes right up against me, lift him to my shoulder using only my arms, then stand straight up without bending my back at all.

It worked really well!

It was a little more difficult to put him down when he was

sleeping, because after I slid him down the front of my body to the mattress I had to push him away from the edge of the bed without waking him up. Like a rope, he was easier to pull than to push. I was always very aware of how strange this new routine would look if anyone was watching, and it made me chuckle every time.

Even as Chris started crawling, my back remained chronically swollen and sore. I was so sensitive that I could no longer tolerate the chiropractic treatment that had provided relief in the past. Conservative measures such as ice and over-the-counter pain medication recommended by my primary care doctor were no longer effective, and I pressed for a more aggressive approach. He referred me to a spine surgeon.

At the spine surgeon's office I paced around the small exam room while I waited for the doctor, glancing at the anatomical posters on the walls and little spine models on the countertops. My back was stiff and tender, and I wanted to wait as long as possible before climbing onto the hard exam table. I didn't get too close to the almost life-size skeleton swaying on a portable stand from a bolt in his head. He was kinda creepy.

The doctor, a mild-mannered man in his forties with short black hair and stylish, thick- framed glasses, entered the room and introduced himself with a gentle handshake. He wrote a couple of notes on a piece of paper clipped to the inside of a manila folder as I described my symptoms, and then asked me to lay back on the exam table so he could perform some tests.

He first lifted my legs into a number of different positions to gauge my response. He then measured the strength on each side of my body by holding my feet while I pushed and pulled his hands. He assessed my ability to walk on my toes and heels, and, finally, looked for unusual curvature as I leaned forward touching my toes.

The doctor's slight nods during the assessment made me feel like he understood what was causing my pain, but he didn't give anything away. I was anxious to hear what he thought about my condition and to find out what treatment he would recommend. I was ready to get back to normal. I needed to sleep, and wanted to be able to play with the kids.

When we were done with the tests, my back ached and burned as I stood on wobbly legs and looked at him expectantly. He said he needed additional information and handed me an order for an MRI.

I had the MRI, then returned to the spine surgeon to find out the results. I was in the same exam room studying a poster of back muscles when the doctor walked in with a disc in his hand. He sat on a stool and loaded the disc into a computer on a small work-top, then scrolled through a number of file names until he found what he was looking for. He clicked on it, and a black-and- white image that looked like an X-ray popped onto a screen just below eye level on the wall. I hunched over to see it while he looked up from the desk.

"This is why you are feeling pain. Do you see here?" he said, moving his computer mouse to point to an area near the middle of the screen. "These discs are compressed and degenerated."

Noticing my blank look, he picked up a spine model and flexed it from side to side. "See how these healthy discs are thick and soft? They are shock absorbers for your back. When you bend and twist they absorb the movement and protect the nerves in your spine." He touched several of the elastic projections sticking out a couple of inches from each section of the spine like tree branches.

He then returned to the MRI image and moved his mouse around, tracing three dark, jagged-looking spaces between blocky sections of bone.

"Your discs are damaged and are not able to do their job. They are thin and rigid, and this entire area is irritated and inflamed."

He emphasized his point by pushing his thumb into a spot in my lower back to the right of my spine, and nearly sent me through the roof.

13

"Wow!" I yelped, not only out of surprise and in response to the sharp pain, but also out of respect for his ability to find that exact spot through my clothes on his first try.

"I would like for you to go to physical therapy," he said, as he wrote something unintelligible on a prescription pad.

I signed on for the prescribed therapy sessions, three times each week for six weeks. My therapist met me in the lobby for the first session, then escorted me to a small office for an initial assessment. She was in her twenties with a bouncy blond ponytail, and wore khakis with a navy blue polo shirt. She looked athletic and I wanted to ask her if she played any sports, but she was very focused on preparing a plan and getting started with my treatment. She said we would conduct another assessment at the end of the six weeks so she could report my progress to my doctor.

I touched my toes and practiced standing up from a chair while she took measurements and notes. She said she had reviewed information provided by my spine surgeon and was ready to get me started in the gym.

When she opened the door to the therapy center, I stopped to take it all in. Patients and therapists bustled around the huge open space that made up most of the top floor of the office building. Large windows and clear white lights brightened the room. Exercise bikes and treadmills stood side by side on the far wall, with racks of weights in each corner. Straps hung from the ceiling in the middle of the room, and several big pieces of equipment were scattered throughout. On the left was a large wooden structure with sturdy handrails that looked like a bridge. Three steps in the front led to a wide platform, then a long ramp sloped down the back. To the right was a metal replica of the front half of a car. Bright floor mats and a wide variety of colorful balls in the middle of the room reminded me of a children's playground.

My therapist led me to a mat and showed me a number of exercises designed to strengthen and relax the muscles around my spine. I liked the side twists where I lay on my back with my knees bent and feet flat on the floor, then dropped both legs to one side and the other by twisting only from the waist. I could feel a nice stretch in my lower back during that one.

Most of the other exercises, though, required more spine movement and were very uncomfortable. My least favorite was the cat/cow, where I arched my back like a cat, then sagged like a cow while on my hands and knees. The cat part was okay, but when I dropped my stomach toward the floor for the cow sag, my body jerked back to a neutral position in protest.

I was able to complete several repetitions of the bridge exercise, where I started on my back with my feet flat on the floor, then lifted my hips in the air. That motion was okay as long as I didn't push my hips too far forward. But when I rolled onto my stomach for the first cobra stretch, I was beginning to feel increased pressure in my back and a deep, sickening pain. I straightened my arms to raise my upper body while my hips and legs remained flat on the floor as instructed, and immediately felt a sharp pain through my spine. I dropped my chest to the floor while I tried to catch my breath. I felt light-headed.

"Nice job!" the therapist told me at the end of the first session as she walked me to the door. "You will feel a little more sore than usual, since you have been protecting your back and not exercising the muscles. Our activities today stressed the muscles in a good way, and the pain you'll feel at first indicates progress. It's good pain! The muscles will strengthen and heal. Take some Advil and put ice on your back when you get home if you have any discomfort."

I wanted to believe her and accept that the pain I felt was good, but I felt nauseated and my legs felt weak as I gingerly inched through the building. I was barely able to push the gas and brake pedals as I drove home.

Early in the third therapy session I was struggling to complete half the number of exercises I did during the first session because of pain and pressure in my back. I tried my best to continue, but was shaking and covered in sweat.

"Don't worry, it's normal to have setbacks," the therapist told me as she led me to a padded treatment table in a dark corner at the back of the room. I thought she sounded disappointed, but I might've imagined that.

An elderly woman on a matching table five feet away lay on her back while a therapist raised the woman's arm above her head over and over and pressed gently into her shoulder. Their conversation about the woman's young grandson insisting on carrying her purse since her shoulder surgery made me smile and was a welcome distraction from the disappointment I felt about my progress. I was going in the wrong direction and was beginning to worry that therapy was not going to help my condition.

The therapist positioned me on my stomach with a pillow under my head. She used tongs to pull a quilted-looking pad out of steaming hot water then placed it on a towel on my lower back. The pad was about twelve by eighteen inches, heavy, hot, and felt wonderful. For fifteen minutes I stayed there with my eyes closed, soothed by the conversation next to me and the moist heat.

By the end of the second week of therapy I was miserable. I could hardly walk because of pain and cramping, and my back was so sensitive the pressure from the mat took my breath away. I trembled and became nauseous almost immediately when I attempted the exercises, and spent increasingly more time on the treatment table with a heat pack on my back.

My therapist insisted that the entire series of sessions was necessary for maximum benefit, so I completed the six-week commitment. By the end my back was so weak and raw I couldn't walk and breathe at the same time. My feet felt like heavy weights, and when I tried to lift them a stabbing pain clamped the muscles in my back. My back burned and was extremely sore to the touch, like an infected wound.

Chapter Four

RELIEF

I returned to my spine surgeon to report the outcome of therapy and to find out what was next to help me return to my normal level of physical activity. In the same small exam room, I studied the thick pink discs between the vertebrae of a little spine model on the counter, and wondered how he would fix my damaged discs. Maybe I needed surgery? That sounded scary, but I thought it must've been pretty routine for a spine surgeon.

I was standing with my knees bent and hands on my thighs to try to relieve a sudden cramp in my back when the doctor opened the door and took a step into the room. He stopped and looked at me curiously.

"Therapy really irritated my back," I said, with a grimace and a little grunt as my breath caught in my throat during a strong spasm. "It's cramping all the time. Makes the pain so much worse."

He opened my file and flipped through a few pages while I carefully climbed onto the table. For a minute or two I watched him read and wondered what the therapist wrote in her note to him, then squirmed and shifted in an attempt to find a comfortable position while I waited for him to look up and tell me our next steps.

"I'm sorry that didn't help you," he said as he jotted something in the folder. "There is nothing else I can do."

I flinched. *What??*

I considered him, then the rest of the room. Wasn't he a spine specialist? How could he not help me?

I was ready to do something, to try anything. I was not ready to accept that the exhausting, sickening pain that clouded every minute of my day and night was a permanent part of my life.

He closed the folder and watched me for a minute before he calmly continued. "You have to adjust your lifestyle to avoid activities that irritate your back."

I was torn between wanting to cry and wanting to scream. All activities irritated my back! I was constantly tired and grumpy, guarded and tentative. Not at all the excited and adventurous parent I wanted to be for my kids. I cringed as I remembered snapping at Kenny the day before when he bumped into me on the driveway while roller-skating, sending a bolt of intense pain through my spine. His lively chatter stopped immediately and his face dropped in surprise as I yelled at him to be more careful.

I wanted to be a patient and empathetic mother. Was that hope gone?

With a big lump in my throat I said, "There must be something we can do."

"I'm sorry," he said. "What you do depends on the quality of life you would like to have. You can engage in whatever activities you want. But you will have to live with the pain."

He gave me a weak smile, then left the room.

Quality of life? I was in my early thirties with three small children. What quality of life did I have if I avoided all activities that caused pain?

I hadn't realized how hopeful I was when I arrived for the appointment, but was suddenly aware of how devastated I felt by the finality of the doctor's words. There was nothing he could do. I rolled off the table and went home, imagining a life where I would have to calculate every move and would never be eager to play with the kids.

After Gretchen and Kenny were born, I exercised at home three or more days a week, running on a treadmill or following an aerobics video. On Tuesdays and Thursdays if Phil was in town I met a group of my friends for an early morning jog while the rest of the house was still sleeping.

Even months after completing therapy, I was no longer able to do any of those things. No matter how careful I was, my back was not getting better. I gave away my exercise videos and told my friends to go on without me.

I woke up early on jogging days out of habit, and looked out the window at my friends talking on the sidewalk as they waited for everyone to arrive. I was reminded of sitting in the dugout with my high school softball team wearing a brace on my leg, out for the season, after I had torn ligaments in my ankle. At first I was still part of the team. I sat on the same bench, wearing the same jersey, and shouting the same cheers. But very quickly I became an outsider. The team inched farther away each time I didn't run out to take the field. Eventually my teammates no longer turned to me on the bench, and I became no different than a spectator in the stands.

As I watched my friends jog away, I knew they would soon stop looking at my house to see if a light was on. They would eventually start meeting in front of someone else's house. But this time I would not start over next season like nothing had happened. I was out of the game for good.

Who was I if not physically active and physically competitive? I wasn't someone who moved cautiously, afraid of being hurt!

I resolved to reduce my pain so I could return to my normal life as much as possible by building accommodations into my daily activities. I slept flat on my back on the floor with a pillow under my knees so I could keep my spine perfectly straight to avoid painful spasms in the middle of the night. I slid a pillow behind my back when I drove a car to fill the gap at the base of the seat and put a soft wedge cushion on my chair at work to avoid pressure on my spine. I stopped wearing high-heeled shoes because they were unstable, and started walking slightly on my toes to avoid the jarring pain caused by my heels hitting the floor. I no longer sat on the floor to play games with the kids or curled up on soft mattresses to read stories at bedtime.

Unsatisfied with my new habits and unwilling to give up on my desire for a more active lifestyle, I returned to my primary care doctor. He practiced with a group of other doctors, and the large, modern office was always very busy. In the packed waiting room I could only find a tiny seat in the "kid zone" below a television blaring *Nickelodeon* cartoons. The little wooden chair and my overly folded knees immediately sent my back into spasms. I stood and slowly shuffled around the crowded room, drawing a few concerned glances from other patients.

In the exam room I sat on a cushioned chair next to a small computer counter as a nurse leaned over the keyboard on a stool beside me, asking about current medications and symptoms. She took my temperature with an electronic ear thermometer and my blood pressure the old-fashioned way, with a hand pump and a stethoscope, then left.

The doctor entered immediately and plopped down in front of the computer. He was in his thirties, tall and slim with curly brown hair, and wore a casual button-down shirt with khakis. I explained the reason for my visit while he reviewed my history. He asked me to move to the table, where he listened to my heart, then looked in my ears and mouth.

"I want you to see a rheumatologist," he said, with no further explanation.

He went out and came back with a sheet of paper that had been copied so many times the information was almost illegible, then circled one of three names.

I didn't really know what a rheumatologist was, but I was willing to do anything that moved me in a positive direction.

The rheumatologist's office was only about fifteen minutes from home, but in an area I'd never been to before. On the way, I passed a beautiful lake surrounded by a variety of little shops and restaurants and made a note to come back with Phil and the kids.

Unlike my primary care doctor's office, which was bright and fresh, the rheumatologist was in a medical building with dark hallways, peeling wallpaper, and stained carpet. Once in his suite I was relieved to find it neat and clean. The furniture was a little dated and it smelled like an old bookstore, but it did not feel neglected.

The rheumatologist practiced alone, so there were only a couple of people in the quiet waiting area. No television, no kids, no talking. Just a few faces buried in magazines. I focused on completing my new-patient forms, and tried to get comfortable on the hard wooden chair while I waited for my turn. Once the waiting room was empty and my name was called, I was met at the door by the middle-aged male doctor in a worn white coat.

The doctor led me to a small room and helped me onto the exam table. With a soft voice and no sense of urgency he reviewed my forms out loud, hesitating and looking up at me periodically for confirmation. He drew my blood himself, and said we would review results and course of action at a follow-up visit.

When I returned, the office was busier and my interaction with the doctor felt rushed. He escorted me out of the crowded lobby and through the small hallway in the back, stopping outside the third closed exam room door. He pushed a couple of pages of blood test results in my hand and pointed out a section of numbers.

"You have rheumatoid arthritis," he said, "an autoimmune disease that causes your body to attack itself. The result is systemic inflammation and painful joints, including your spine."

He put his hand on my shoulder to guide me back toward the waiting room as he said, "There is no cure; you will suffer from the disease for the rest of your life."

He stopped at the door to the lobby and wrote out two prescriptions on a pad, then tore them off and handed them to me. As he opened the door he said, "Daily medications will stop the self-destruction and will be very effective in addressing your symptoms.

I walked out of his office in a daze, prescriptions in hand, without asking any questions. While I was encouraged by his confidence in the treatment, I was confused by the unexpected identification of what sounded like a serious condition. Plus, on my way out, I noticed that the waiting room was full of people who looked like my grandparents. Were all of his patients more than twice my age?

I trusted my primary care doctor and he recommended this rheumatologist, so I reasoned that the diagnosis and treatment must have been appropriate. But why were all the patients so much older than I was? Was it unusual for me to have this disorder at age thirty-four?

In the car I reviewed my blood test results, which reported a very high level of antinuclear antibodies (ANA), which apparently indicated autoimmune disease. The reference information at the bottom of the page stated that high levels of ANA were "often noted in older individuals and in patients with a diversity of non-rheumatologic complaints."

The results were pretty clear, but the typical patient didn't sound like me, so this information confused me further.

The "disease" label continued to disturb me as I filled my prescriptions and began my medication regimen. I didn't know anyone with a disease diagnosis, and I'd never heard of autoimmune disease. Wouldn't I have other symptoms if I had a serious chronic illness?

I felt fine other than my back pain. I'd had a few surgeries, but nothing I thought was unusual at the time. There were two operations on my jaw in college because it sometimes slipped sideways when I chewed and would get stuck if I opened my mouth too widely. Both of my knees had been scoped twice to remove damaged cartilage, and I'd had shoulder surgery to address painful grinding in the joint when I rotated my arm. Each issue was explained away as the result of normal wear and tear, overuse, or injury. Considering the possible impact of inflammatory disease on my joints, I wondered if rheumatoid arthritis was actually the cause.

I easily fell into my new routine of taking daily medications to suppress my immune system and reduce inflammation, and checking in with the rheumatologist every few months. The routine bloodwork almost always indicated a low white blood cell count, requiring the tests to be repeated several times to achieve a marginally normal result. The doctor never expressed any concern, and I didn't think anything about it.

I was elated to discover that the treatment reduced my back pain to a functional level. I still couldn't twist or bend without pain, but the constant burning and cramping were gone. As long as I maintained my cautious lifestyle, my base level pain was mild and tolerable.

I was working part time, writing scientific reports or planning experiments during my couple of days at work each week and when I could find an hour or two at home.

Gretchen, now in first grade, behaved like a young executive. She had consistently popped out of bed on time since the first day of kindergarten when she told me, "I have an alarm clock. I don't need you to wake me up for school." I wasn't sure if she felt strongly about her independence or just didn't trust me to get it right.

Every day after school, Gret lined up her stuffed animals and gathered her little brothers for "old-time school," where she taught them a version of whatever she had learned that day. There were bells and report cards and snacks, and the boys seemed to respect their enthusiastic teacher. I appreciated the distraction after a full day of work or a day at home with two active boys, especially when my back was sore or tight and I needed a few minutes to rest.

My arthritis occasionally "flared up" without warning, and my pain escalated to an unbearable level far beyond what I had experienced before. When this happened I would lie with my back flat on the floor and my feet up on the couch or a chair. I couldn't move or sleep, sometimes for several days. Just taking a deep breath during these episodes caused severe muscle spasms, and a sneeze or cough resulted in the most incredible pain I had ever experienced. If I was able to get myself off the floor, I could drop by the rheumatologist's office for pain-killing injections directly into the muscles of my lower back. The doctor never seemed surprised to see me off-cycle and was not alarmed by these events. I was simply thankful that the injections provided a few hours of complete pain relief so I could rest.

Chapter Five

A SHOCK

During an annual physical exam when I was thirty-five, my doctor told me that my insurance would pay for one mammogram between ages thirty-five and forty and that I should take advantage of it. I left the office thinking that I should get the mammogram sometime before I turned forty, and then did nothing. I was picking up more hours at work and so busy shuffling the kids from one activity to another I didn't prioritize anything that wasn't urgent. Gretchen and Kenny played soccer and took swimming lessons, and Chris was in a class at a children's gym. We constantly ran from one activity to the next.

At my annual exam when I was thirty-six, the doctor very gently explained that I should go for the mammogram at the earliest time possible (last year, you dummy), so there would be a baseline for comparison when I turned forty. I scheduled an appointment.

As a relatively modest person with minimal experience exposing and discussing my breasts in the company of strangers, I was apprehensive about my first mammogram. I scheduled the exam late in the afternoon so I could work most of the day and still pick the kids up on time from daycare afterward.

Traffic was slow due to rain, but I pulled into the medical complex at exactly my appointment time. Initially relieved, I was quickly disappointed. Rather than a single office building, I found a series of identical one-story brick structures with big numbers or letters on the front. There were multiple entrances and internal roadways, similar to an apartment complex. I wound around looking for my number, becoming more anxious with every minute that passed. I finally found it, but could not find a place to park. Eventually I pulled into a spot five buildings away and ran back through the rain.

I was instructed not to wear deodorant on the day of the procedure, and as I ran I became concerned that all my rushing and the sprint from my car in a heavy raincoat was going to create an offensive situation for whoever was going to be performing the exam. I jerked open the door to the nondescript structure and stepped into a small entryway between the external and an open internal door, brushing the water off my pants and shaking my raincoat.

I looked up and immediately froze. I had never seen such a beautiful, welcoming waiting area. Couches and chairs with dark brown wooden legs and wide forest green and burgundy stripes filled the room. Large, clear glass bowls of pink-wrapped candies, neatly organized magazines, bold flowers arrangements, and racks of perfectly aligned brochures covered the polished tabletops. Huge Monet-like prints hung on the walls, so close together their frames nearly touched.

I walked toward the receptionist. "I'm so sorry to be late. I was held up at work and there was traffic, then I couldn't find the building or a place to park."

"Don't worry, it's fine," she said pleasantly, taking my driver's license, insurance card, and a soggy order for the procedure.

I turned to find a seat, and realized the room seemed remarkably . . . feminine. The genuine warmth I felt from the other women as they looked up from their magazines gave me a surprising sense of small-town camaraderie I had not experienced since leaving Tennessee more than ten years earlier.

My name was called almost immediately and I followed someone in scrubs through an inner door. We stopped at the entrance to a second waiting room that looked very similar to the first, but was smaller.

Instructions came at me in a rush. "Go into any empty changing room. Take off everything from the waist up. You don't have any deodorant on, right? Great. If you do, use these wipes to remove it. Leave your clothes in the dressing room. Nobody will bother them. Bring your purse and any valuables. Take off this necklace. You can leave on the earrings. Put on a gown open to the front. You can pick one up here. Have a seat and someone will be right in to get you."

I picked up a gown and couple of wipe packets from a countertop inside the door, then looked down the row of tiny dressing rooms that lined the side wall of the waiting area. I found an open curtain toward the middle of the room and slipped inside. A small mirror hung on the left side, and a couple of clothes hooks on the right. A narrow shelf was tacked to the back wall.

The curtain was too small to close completely, and I felt self-conscious about changing with women sitting just a few feet away. I turned my back and quickly undressed, passing a wipe over each arm pit to address my concerns about odor. I pulled on a gown and struggled to keep it from hanging open even with the strings tied. Giving up, I exited the dressing room while self-consciously holding the gown closed with one hand. I slid into a high-back chair in the far corner of the room and chuckled as I noticed several other women clutching the tops of their gowns with one hand as they flipped through magazines with the other.

My name was again called pretty quickly, and the procedure was pretty unremarkable. It was a little awkward with the unfamiliar pulling, squishing, and standing around bare-chested, but the technician was very professional and friendly. Before I had time to think much about it, I was back in the changing room getting dressed to go home.

The next week I received a call from the imaging center. The radiologist was unable to see one area of my right breast well enough for a thorough evaluation and wanted me to come in to repeat the procedure.

No problem. I scheduled an early appointment the following week so I could stop by on my way to work.

I followed the same routine as before, but was asked to remain in my gown in the small waiting room after the mammogram while the radiologist reviewed the images. I sat in the high- back chair holding my gown closed and prepared a quick mental "to do" list for my day. I needed to review client requirements for a project meeting at noon, when we would discuss plans to address significant changes to our standard testing protocol. At two o'clock I was joining a group interview for a new scientist and should probably prepare some questions.

Suddenly a technician appeared in front of me, interrupting my thoughts. She led me out of the waiting room and explained that the radiologist wanted to perform a sonogram to further evaluate the unclear area, which was not resolved by the second mammogram.

Okay, I thought, with a quick glance at my watch. *If this doesn't take too long I will still be on schedule.*

The technician walked me into a dark room, where a professional-looking woman in a lab coat, the radiologist, was setting up sonogram equipment. She was small and slender with dark hair gathered neatly into a wide clip halfway down her neck. Her back was to the door as she pushed buttons and rearranged cords on her big rolling cart. The technician dropped my gown off my shoulders so it hung around my waist, and helped me lay back onto the narrow exam table next to the machine. Without a word the radiologist squirted warm gel onto my skin, then pressed the sonogram wand firmly into my breast. She studied the screen and looked over at me when necessary to reposition the wand or add more gel.

"Can you see what you need?" I asked. "Are you getting a better image than you had before?"

No answer.

"What do you see?" I asked.

No response. I gave up.

After a few minutes she carefully wiped gel off the wand and returned it to its holder on the side of the cart. She clicked on a keyboard and dragged a cursor across the screen as I lay bare-chested on the table. She created dots and lines very similar to sonograms I had experienced during pregnancy to measure the baby's size.

The radiologist abruptly leaned over and wiped the gel off my chest with a soft, warm towel. She put her hand out to grasp mine and pulled me up to a sitting position. I fumbled with the crumpled gown to cover my chest.

"There is an area of your breast that is highly indicative of breast cancer," she said. "Who is your surgeon?"

Immediately I was very embarrassed for her.

My surgeon? Breast cancer? How ridiculous! I'm on my way to work. I don't have a surgeon. I'm only thirty-six years old!

I stopped struggling to cover myself and dropped my gown as she and the technician walked out. I stared, stunned, at the screen of the ultrasound machine. It looked like a starlit sky, her lines indicating constellations.

The radiologist quickly returned. I sat bare-chested in the dark, my hands limp on my lap. She flipped on the light and held out a phone to me. "It's your doctor."

"Hello?" I said.

"Hi," my doctor said. "Listen, I know what's going on right now is really scary, but it doesn't mean anything until you have a biopsy. I know a wonderful surgeon who will take great care of you. I'm going to call him as soon as I get off the phone with you, then I will call you back and tell you what happens next. Okay?"

My doctor. On the phone. Immediately available to talk to me?

I handed the phone back to the radiologist and studied her. She put a brochure in my hand that said something like "So you have cancer" and walked out the door. I started to shake.

I slid off the table and pulled the gown loosely over my shoulders like a jacket, making no effort to cover my exposed stomach. I brushed past women with their magazines in the small waiting area. I felt like I was on another planet. My body seemed to be moving without conscious thought, and I was numb all over. I dressed, took my necklace from a hook and dropped it into the pocket of my overcoat, then walked straight out the door.

It was a rainy and cool October day. I wandered aimlessly through the maze of short brown buildings, watching the rain bounce off tiny white pebbles in the sidewalk. I felt sick.

After a while I sat on a couple of steps in the sidewalk and called Phil. Crying softly and shaking violently, I told him everything that had just happened. Words tumbled out of my mouth, but I didn't feel like I was saying them. Everything was a fuzzy blur except for those little white pebbles.

I don't remember driving home or much about the rest of that week. Phil and I researched breast cancer types and survival rates, and tried hard to get used to the idea that something deadly was growing inside my body.

Mechanically, with no emotion other than complete shock, I met with a surgeon and scheduled a biopsy. I waited for the minor procedure for two weeks and went through the motions of dropping off and picking up the kids, feeding them, bathing them, reading to them, and putting them to bed. They had birthdays over the summer and were seven, five, and two years old.

I realized with paralyzing desperation that they probably would not remember me if I died while they were so young. I imagined what their lives would be like growing up without a mother. I was raised with a big, extended family and had enjoyed plenty of love and support throughout my life. We shared the most routine activities and life's greatest achievements and failures with complete openness and trust. I wanted to provide the same sense of unconditional love for the kids.

We had moved away from my hometown and big family before the kids were born. Phil's father was the only relative within three hundred miles. I couldn't bear to think of the pressure on Phil and Boppa to provide everything the children needed, or the thought of the kids feeling sad or alone.

They were so happy and innocent. I couldn't leave them!

The biopsy was a minor, routine procedure. I knew we needed the pathology results before a definite diagnosis, but Phil and I were told that the surgeon was confident it was cancer. He'd found a golf ball-size black, slimy tumor deep in the center of my breast. Apparently the look and feel of the tissue were very telling.

Because I was groggy from anesthesia, I couldn't really process the information Phil gave me as we drove home. I kept asking again and again, "So it's cancer?"

The anesthesia wore off and the truth began to sink in. I had cancer. Now, with no hope of a different outcome, I went through the motions of my day but felt detached. I watched the kids play and my coworkers discuss projects just as they had done only weeks before. But I was an observer. I was back in the softball dugout with my injured ankle, but this time the game I was watching was my life. I was no longer a key player, and didn't know if I ever would be again. I felt like I was standing in an underground tunnel while the world carried on as usual around me, not noticing that I was there, alone in the dark.

Well-intentioned friends told me everything was going to be fine, but that statement devastated me. Everything was not fine, and there was a real possibility it was going to get much worse. I needed to be able to cry and scream and express my worst fears. Whenever someone said "fine" I felt forced to live a lie, to pretend that everything was okay even as I crumbled inside. By avoiding the truth and pretending everything was okay, I felt like the people around me were telling me we had no relationship if I could not be the person they knew before. I was pretty sure that person was gone.

I stared at myself in the mirror with a strange sense of separation. Stitched, bruised yellow and green, and oddly pitted where tissue had been removed, the breast did not seem to belong to me. I was a stranger in my own body.

How could my body be destructing me when I didn't even know anything was wrong? What black, slimy toxin remained inside, invading and destroying my life? Was it spreading through my body now, consuming me as I watched helplessly? Could I stop it? Was this the beginning of the end for me?

A few days after the biopsy I met with my surgeon to review pathology results and discuss next steps. He explained that several types of cancer cells were identified by the pathologist, some very aggressive. I needed surgery to remove the cancerous tissue. I could choose a total mastectomy to remove my entire breast, or a breast-sparing partial mastectomy followed by radiation to kill any remaining cancer cells.

I was terrified by the thought of leaving cancer cells in my body and did not want to live in constant fear that it could be spreading undetected. I elected a total mastectomy. The procedure would be in two weeks.

I scheduled appointments with a plastic surgeon and an oncologist with dread, unnerved by the notion that more people would examine my breast and discuss my cancer. What I really wanted to do was curl into a ball and pretend that the previous weeks had never happened.

I stood in front of the plastic surgeon in a large exam room wearing nothing from the waist up, chilled not only by the cool temperature of the room but also by my discomfort as she moved around me, casually touching and considering my breasts . She was tall and attractive, with stunning green eyes and stylish shoulder-length brown hair. I was intimidated by her energy and confidence. I folded my arms across my bare chest, mortified, as she crossed the room and rummaged through my clothes, pulling out my old, worn bra. Was there no end to my loss of dignity?

"You can use this after your surgery since it doesn't have an underwire, but it won't fit very well," she said as she closely inspected my dated undergarment. "Sports bras and camisoles will be much more comfortable. You need to buy a bunch before your operation."

I walked to the opposite side of the room and took a long white robe off a hook, pulling it on as the doctor tossed my bra back onto the chair with my blouse.

"Breast reconstruction can be performed at the same time as the mastectomy," she said, "saving you the trouble of another operation down the road. I've worked with your surgeon many times before. We will be in the operating room together. He will remove your breast and I will immediately create a new one."

All I wanted to do was go home. I was uncomfortable, embarrassed, and not at all concerned about my appearance after surgery. My throat was tight and I thought I might cry. I pulled the plush robe more snuggly around myself and whispered, "I can't think about this right now. I'll have to come back sometime later."

The doctor asked me to get dressed and meet her outside the room. We sat in a hallway waiting area in chairs that backed to a wall with high windows. Between us was a small table covered with information about breast reconstruction. She patiently watched me scan the brochures and photo albums as I pushed my hands deep into my coat pockets, not ready to enter this new world.

She opened an album and offered it to me. "Many patients feel better when they see a more naturally shaped breast in the mirror after surgery, rather than the unfamiliar look of a flat chest."

I'd learned from my general surgeon that performing a mastectomy is almost like scooping ice cream. The skin is pulled forward, and the entire breast is scooped out from behind. The idea is to lift out all the breast tissue together and not spill any cancer cells back into the body. I understood this general concept, but I had not really considered how my body would actually look after this type of surgery.

I took the album and understood immediately. There were photos of women who had chosen reconstruction, and photos of women who had not. The shape did make a huge difference. I agreed that I wanted to do something, and we discussed the pros and cons of creating a breast using flaps of skin from my body versus artificial implants. I ultimately agreed to simultaneous reconstruction with a silicone implant. We selected the size of my new breast.

I returned to the photos resting in my lap and asked weakly, "Where are the nipples?"

"They are removed with the breast tissue when a total mastectomy is performed," she explained. "I can create one for you a few months after your surgery. It's kinda like origami. Small strips of skin are cut from the chest and then twisted together. It's a very minor procedure. Once it heals, tattooing creates the desired color. I have a guy I recommend. He's very good and has a private room just for this."

An album of photos labeled "nipples" showed impressive results. Long, slanted scars across the breasts were not nearly as startling with a realistic-looking nipple in the center.

My gaze froze on the pictures in front of me.

She gently took the album away and suggested we revisit the topic in a few weeks. On my way out she handed me a reminder card with the date and time of my follow-up visit after surgery.

I started to protest, thinking that I needed to check my calendar first. But then I realized that I had nothing else to work around.

There would be no work, no other commitments. My cancer was now my life. I stood in the entryway of the medical building, trying to rally up the strength to drive home.

Chapter Six

NEW PERSPECTIVE

I arrived for my appointment with the oncologist feeling weary and anxious. I didn't know what role she played in my treatment so was unsure what to expect. Was I going to receive more bad news about my cancer? Would there be a humiliating exam or a painful procedure?

The doctor was one of the best in the region, and her waiting room was packed full of patients of every age and at every stage of treatment. Some looked just as wide-eyed and scared as I was; others appeared more resigned and defeated.

I was struck immediately by the atmosphere. I didn't feel support among a group of people facing similar life-changing diagnoses, but instead a strong sense of individuality and survival. A quick glance around the room filled me with fear and deep anguish. A young man clearly at the end of his life with gray skin hanging from a shockingly thin frame shuffled weakly toward the exit, assisted by a man and a woman who appeared to be his parents. A bald woman with thin clear tubes protruding unnaturally from her chest and neck moved toward the back offices, assisted by her children.

I realized that none of us had the energy to consider what others around us might be going through or the courage to face our worst fears playing out through the lives of others right in front of us. Joining the crowd, I kept my head down and waited for my name to be called.

My visit with the oncologist was very brief. She reviewed my medical history and the biopsy pathology report as I sat in front of the cluttered desk in her office.

"You don't have any risk factors," she said, "but you sure as hell have breast cancer!"

She was very kind and reassuring, and told me there was nothing for me to do until after the mastectomy. New pathology of the removed tissue would determine our next steps.

I told the kids that I would be having surgery, but nothing about the cancer. They were too young to comprehend the significance of what I was facing, and I couldn't see a good reason to explain it to them any sooner than absolutely necessary. I didn't have the strength to take the emotional journey with them or to comfort them once they understood the situation.

I simply told them I would be in the hospital for a few days and sore when I came home. They were excited that Phil's brother and my father were coming to visit and would be spending time with them, and thought nothing more about it.

I was surprised but thankful that they didn't sense my trepidation, and kept my secret from them at the expense of feeling like a fraud. I acted like I would always be there for them when I really didn't believe that was true. But maintaining their carefree lives as long as possible felt like a worthy goal, and losing myself in their untroubled world provided a desperately needed respite from the nightmare I was living.

As the surgery date drew closer I gained businesslike energy. I began to think practically and logistically about what the next few weeks would be like rather than focusing on what the rest of my life might be like. Just as I had done during late pregnancy with each of the kids, I cleaned and overstocked supplies knowing that I would be unable to shop or take care of the house for a few weeks at least. At work I tried to wrap up what I could and hand off what I could not, not knowing when I would return.

The mastectomy was scheduled for Monday, November 12. Several times I checked my overnight bag and the children's clothes laid out for the next three days. I made sure there were enough diapers, and milk in the refrigerator.

My surgery was the same day as Kenny's kindergarten fall concert, a school tradition to celebrate several months of holidays. He had been rehearsing, making artwork, and preparing his outfit for weeks. Kenny was a morning kindergartener, so his performance was scheduled early in the school day. This was perfect for me, since my surgery was scheduled later. I would be able to attend.

Dozens of parents talked and laughed as we filed into the small gymnasium. Phil and I walked to the top of the bleachers, where I could lean back against the wall, or stand if my back began to cramp. We snapped pictures of the adorable kindergarteners wearing colorful headbands of construction paper leaves and shaking tambourines. It was over quickly, and the children lined up to walk back to their classrooms.

Tears rolled down my cheeks as I waved good-bye to Kenny from across the room.

The idea of surgery didn't upset me. I was just completely devastated by the thought that this was the beginning of something that would destroy his sweet innocence. I couldn't imagine a scenario where the kids wouldn't be affected, even by successful treatment.

Would I be able to take care of them? Could I manage even my own life? Would I be a burden? Would I spend the rest of my life and all my energy fighting this disease?

I was going to die of a broken heart if I continued to think this way. I passed through the crowd of my friends and neighbors with my head down, walked home to wash off my makeup and take off my wedding ring, then left for the hospital.

I checked in and took a seat in the huge waiting room packed with people. Phil was uncharacteristically stoic and quiet as he sat down next to me and focused on the floor. Even during a difficult fifteen-hour labor before Gretchen was born he'd laughed and joked, trying to lighten the mood. Now he was serious and withdrawn, clearly struggling with his own thoughts about our future.

Waiting and worrying were exhausting, and I was ready to move forward regardless of what was ahead. A nurse called my name and led us to a large room with rows of hospital beds on each side, separated by curtains. The area was loud and busy, with beeping machines and doctors and nurses bustling around.

The nurse stopped at a bed near the middle of the room between two other patients. One was an older man snoring loudly, and the other was a young woman reading a paperback. The nurse handed me a gown and socks, then asked me to change as she pulled the curtain closed. The gown was exactly like the one I wore for my mammogram only a few short weeks earlier. It seemed like a lifetime ago.

I pulled on the gown and remembered the woman I had been when I learned that I had cancer. I was completely absorbed in my daily activities, only focused on getting to work. I hadn't grappled with the fact that one day I would be gone and the world would go on without me. Now, in the preoperative area of the hospital on the day of my mastectomy, I understood very well. I felt a hint of jealousy for earlier me's innocence.

As I climbed onto the bed, the surgeon pulled open the curtain and greeted us with a big smile. I almost didn't recognize him in scrubs and with his thick brown hair tucked neatly inside a surgical cap. He was handsome with a wholesome look, soft-spoken but confident. His calm presence was a sharp contrast to the excited energy all around us and was immediately comforting.

"All ready?" he asked, barely loud enough for me to hear him over stretchers bouncing by.

I nodded.

Moving to my side he said, "Safety procedures require me to mark the surgical site." He removed a marker from his pocket and signed his name on my right breast. "You have to mark it too."

He handed the pen to me. Startled, I asked, "What do I write?"

"It doesn't matter." He noticed my blank look and said, "Just write 'Yes.'"

For some reason I thought this was hilarious. Maybe the stress of the situation caught up with me or maybe I had a strange reaction to the horrible realization that incorrect body parts were removed often enough to require a safety procedure, but I couldn't stop laughing. Phil looked at me like I had truly lost my mind.

With the pen still in hand and a grin on my face, a team of people in scrubs, hats, and masks rushed in, pushed me down the hall and into the operating room, slid my bed against the operating table, and told me to scoot over. The cold table felt very narrow, and I was afraid I would fall off. The team centered me on the table and quickly vanished, their flurry of busy hands and masked faces replaced by a single anesthesiologist looking down on me from above. I started giggling again as he placed a mask over my nose and mouth. He didn't seem to notice. I looked into the bright, round light behind his head.

"I'm going to give you some medicine now to make you sleep," he said.

Immediately, I was out.

I woke up vomiting in tremendous pain in my hospital bed. I couldn't figure out where I was or why my chest felt like it was tearing apart. Unable to take a deep breath, I pawed at the Ace bandages wrapped around my upper body. Someone standing next to me - a nurse, I realized - gently took my hands and told me not to pull at the bandages. She said the surgery went well and that I needed to rest.

I bent over my clenching stomach and retched loudly. I felt like someone was slowly pulling a hot knife through my chest. Sick, confused, and in amazing pain, I suddenly remembered what I was doing there. I had cancer, I might die, my kids and Phil would have to go on without me.

All I could manage to say was, "Am I okay?"

The nurse put a towel on the pool of vomit in my lap. "Someone will be in as soon as possible to help clean you up. We are very busy and short on techs. It might be a while. Please be patient."

After what seemed like hours, my stomach settled down and I took my forearms off my thighs, trying to unfold myself into an upright position. I was cold and uncomfortable but didn't know how to adjust the bed or call for help.

Finally, a different nurse came into my room. I thought she was there to remove the wet towel and sheets, but instead she walked up with a big smile and plopped a cupcake with a Hershey kiss on top onto my bedside table.

"These cupcakes were made for a breast cancer awareness event because they look like boobs," she said.

I started to cry and explained that I was terrified for myself and my family and I didn't know what to do. She looked at me, then at the dozen or so cupcakes remaining in the plastic container. She apologized, explaining that she wasn't really working on my unit and needed to deliver the rest of her cupcakes.

I began to shake. The cupcake nurse stepped out and my nurse returned. She removed the wet linen, helped situate me in the bed, wrapped me in warm blankets, and gave me pain medication. I was quickly asleep.

After three days in the hospital I was sent home with a drain to remove fluids from the wound beneath my bandages. A four-inch-wide bruise covered the center of my chest from my collarbones down to my waist. Apparently the chest muscle lining was scraped as part of the surgical procedure to remove as many cancer cells as possible.

My discharge instructions emphasized that the breast implant had to be aggressively massaged several times a day to prevent scar tissue from forming a hard capsule around it. After passing out during this incredibly painful procedure the first time, I learned to take pain medication and lay on the floor before starting the massage. Even with these precautions I fainted once more at home, and also passed out at the plastic surgeon's office during my follow- up appointment. She removed two-week-old bandages and quickly pulled out the drain tube, then poked and prodded. The next thing I knew I was in a dark room with my feet up and a cold towel on my head.

During my recovery from surgery, friends and neighbors brought food, shuffled kids around, and took up a collection to pay someone to clean my house. When I encountered one of these kindhearted people I could see sympathy in their eyes, but also fear. Was that for me, or were they afraid of the realization that something terrible could happen in their own lives?

Either way, they were clearly much more comfortable exchanging casual pleasantries and discussing logistics than participating in a meaningful conversation. That was fine with me! I was exhausted from weeks of feeling sad and scared, and happy to talk about anything other than my health.

Several people told me I was strong and brave, but I felt neither. Someone who was strong and brave faced their fears with a sense of command. I faced my fears with complete terror. I felt more like someone tumbling around in a giant clothes dryer trying to survive rather than a warrior leading an attack. I hadn't decided to boldly do anything. During what part of all of this did I have a choice?

As the pain decreased and I grew stronger, I became more familiar with my new physical condition. I was still unable to pick up two-year-old Chris, but I was able to use my arms for light tasks.

The muscles on the right side of my chest moved differently than before. Rather than flex smoothly, the muscles' response was delayed and then sudden. They seemed to snap from resting to their new flexed position with no transition. While it wasn't painful, the sensation was quite unnerving.

I started feeling better, but since I wasn't yet back to work and my normal routine I had far too much time to think. No matter how hard I tried to live in the moment and think positively, I was paralyzed by the prospect of a dark future. I wanted to pretend that nothing was wrong and move on, ignoring the need for any further action.

What if I just canceled all future appointments and went back to work, back to my life before all of this happened? None of this seemed real the way my old life did. The moment the radiologist told me I had cancer I felt as if someone threw a bag over everything I knew, pulled a drawstring to close it, and jerked it away from me. I longed for my lost sense of reality.

I didn't feel like I was dying. Did that mean I would be okay, or did everyone feel this way in the beginning? How soon would that feeling change? Should I do something relevant while I had the energy? Start ticking items off a bucket list? Write meaningful letters to each of the kids for them to read when they were grown if I was gone?

Pathology of breast tissue removed during the mastectomy would determine my fate. At the follow-up appointment with my surgeon I would find out if I could return to work and my normal life, even temporarily, or if I would be too sick from the next phase of my treatment to do anything other than get through it. He would tell me how long I had before fighting was all I could do, until I didn't care, until I was gone.

I was ready. I needed to move forward.

I felt weak and extremely vulnerable as I sat in the bright exam room and waited for the surgeon. I wore only a paper vest-like gown on my upper body, and crossed my arms across my chest for warmth and modesty. The small vest didn't come close to closing in the front, and was so short it didn't cover my waistline. Even after becoming a little more accustomed to regular discussion and review of my breasts over the previous weeks, at that moment I felt exceptionally exposed.

The doctor checked my scars and the range of motion in my arm, then asked me to change and meet him in his office.

"You are healing well!" he said, greeting me at his office door with a big smile and a gentle squeeze of my shoulder. "How do you feel?"

I was so focused on what came next I didn't respond. I slid into a chair in front of his desk as he sat down behind it. Still feeling cold though fully dressed and wearing a jacket, I recrossed my arms and slumped forward. I was terrified, and braced myself for the big announcement.

He opened my file on his desk and removed two copies of the new pathology report, handing one to me. I tried to follow along as he reviewed the list of complex medical terms. He pointed out the same multiple types of cancer found by the initial biopsy, emphasizing the aggressive nature of some of them.

I felt like someone was piling weights on my back. The little energy I had was draining from my body. I sunk deeper into my chair.

The doctor's reading slowed as he more thoroughly considered the final pathological diagnosis section at the end of the report.

"A one-millimeter margin of healthy tissue surrounded the cancer that was removed from your body," he said. "Noninvasive."

He put down the paper and looked at me. I stared back, not noticing his pleased and expectant expression. I patiently waited for the part where he would tell me what we do next. How I would lose my hair and be too weak to eat.

Instead he said, "We got it all. You don't need radiation or chemotherapy. No cancer cells remain in your body. You should get a mammogram and schedule an appointment with me every six months. Be sure to bring the actual films rather than just the radiology report so I can -"

Wait, what? No chemo or radiation? I was done??

I didn't even know that was an option! I felt completely disoriented, so focused on finding out when I was going to die that I never considered that I might actually live. I sat up very straight, my heart pounding. I was suddenly full of energy.

I finally noticed that he looked like someone delivering good news, but I still felt cautious. I challenged him to be sure. "I'm sorry, can you say that again? What do we need to do now?"

"You are done," he said with a warm smile. "You had aggressive cancer, but now it's gone. You are not in remission, you are cancer-free. A few more months without surgery and you would've faced a very different prognosis. I will keep an eye on you, but I don't expect any problems."

The next thing I knew I was sitting in my car, giddy with relief. I felt a desperate need to see the kids, to celebrate victory over a battle they didn't even know I was fighting.

Anguish washed over me as I thought of them, my brain not yet able to realize the absence of mortal danger. I started to laugh and resisted a powerful impulse to kneel on the parking lot outside my car and kiss the ground out of gratitude and humility.

I noticed the pathology report in my hand and reread every word. Suddenly I felt extremely guilty that I was abandoning people with cancer who were fighting every day for their lives and giving up everything important to them. Just moments ago they were my people.

Would I simply forget them and everything I had learned? I truly understood what they were going through, at least to a point. Should I now just erase those thoughts and memories and move on, happy to shed such a heavy burden?

Of course, my friends and family would be relieved and anxious to return to normal activities and conversations, but I didn't want that. I wanted to somehow remain changed. I vowed that my scars would serve as a constant reminder of my experience, of the others fighting, and of lives lost. I didn't want to forget.

Once I was home I busied myself with picking up toys and starting laundry as I waited for the kids. My tears flowed freely as I hugged them at the door, surprising both them and me. I explained that I was crying happy tears because the doctor said I was getting better and would be able to play with them more. They accepted this information without a second thought, shared stories of their day, and ran off to play.

Within a few weeks I was back to work and my old routines. While my life appeared to be the same as before, I felt like a different person. My new perspective gave me a calm disposition, and a maturity that I thought must have been as obvious as gray hair and wrinkles.

Many people who were aware of my experience shared their stories about mothers, sisters, wives, aunts, and grandmothers who died from breast cancer, which filled me with pain and suffocating guilt. Why did I survive and these wonderful people, who were so loved and needed, die? No one ever gave me the slightest impression that they were resentful, but I was very aware that others, for no good reason at all, had a very different outcome.

I also knew that the loved ones with a hole in their lives could have just as easily been mine.

Chapter Seven

CHANGES

The following year Phil and I divorced. We were completely different people than we had been when we married fifteen years earlier at age twenty-two. The demands of his job and caring for an aging father consumed his energy, while I was focused on my work, health, and a very busy household. Neither of us prioritized our relationship or each other. We remained friendly and respectful, and focused on the kids. The kids seemed unbothered, more excited about having two homes than troubled by the change in our relationship.

Every six months I visited my surgeon so he could watch for recurrence or problems in the other breast, but there were no issues. I never returned to the rheumatologist. I didn't believe the treatment to control my arthritis pain caused my breast cancer, but I no longer thought taking medication to suppress my immune system was a good idea. I wanted my body's normal process of getting rid of harmful cells to be as strong as possible.

Without the daily medications that had been prescribed by the rheumatologist, my back pain was again out of control. Unwilling to return to a life based on pain avoidance, I doggedly pursued a solution. After another round of spine imaging, over-the-counter medications, and torturous physical therapy, my doctor suggested prescription medications for pain and inflammation. He provided multiple refills for the drugs, along with instructions for taking a non-prescription medication such as Prilosec twice a day to prevent damage to my stomach lining that could result from long-term use of strong anti-inflammatories.

The effectiveness of the new medications was amazing, and far exceeded my hopes for returning to a functional level of activity. I was able to sleep in my bed and could move around normally without worrying that a slight twist of my spine or thump of my foot would send my back into spasms. Why didn't we do this sooner?

I quickly realized that low-impact exercise was tolerable, enabling me to use an elliptical machine and participate in martial arts classes. I was shocked to find that I continued to feel better as the frequency and intensity of my physical activity increased. The doctor was not surprised, explaining that improved blood flow and muscle strength reduced pain and cramping and lessened my nerves' vulnerability to irritation.

At last I was able to be myself with the kids. For the first time since Chris was born I had no emotional or physical issues separating me from them. Cancer no longer clouded our future, and back pain no longer defined my actions. I was whole, and thrilled to have my life back with the kids at the center of my universe. They were full of energy and excited about everything. I easily matched their optimism and passion for life. I felt fantastic, and planned to be around for the next fifty years or more.

The atmosphere in our house was playful and lively. We danced on the kitchen island many evenings to music blasting from a portable CD player. Motown and dance party songs were our favorites, but we threw in an occasional Kidz Bop or Disney CD, depending on who was selecting the music.

We often hiked near our house and rode bikes several miles to the next town for lunch or ice cream. Gret was always a block ahead, pointing out anything of interest and leading the way. Chris rode on a trailer bike attached to mine, and Kenny constantly lagged behind. Kenny was distracted by everything, dropping his bike to check out an interesting rock or animal print in the dirt. Chris's job was to watch Kenny and remind him to pay attention so he wouldn't crash into the back of our bike as he commented on the clouds or landscape.

Kenny still regularly ran into the back of our bike. There was always something more important to him than watching where he was going. Chris was our safety officer and rule keeper. In kindergarten he listened in the morning when the thirty kids in his class called out their lunch orders to send to the cafeteria, then at lunchtime corrected anyone who inappropriately lined up in the hot dog line when they should have been in the chicken nugget line.

The kids helped me put up drywall, paint, and organize the garage. We fenced off a section of the yard and planted a garden that overflowed with pumpkins, strawberries, carrots, onions, tomatoes, and peppers. We constructed a play area in the basement for our pets, including guinea pigs, mice, rabbits, a rat, and a chinchilla. A snake and a lizard were kept safely separated from the other animals in Gret and Kenny's bedrooms.

I had no delusion that my back issues were resolved. I was very aware that the greatly reduced pain and cramping were due to the strong anti-inflammatories I was taking. If I missed a dose, I was back in my old position on the floor with my feet up, lying perfectly still to avoid pain-induced nausea. I was very, very appreciative of the effect this wonder drug was having on my life.

I was much more comfortable in the car, and we often made the twelve-hour drive to visit my family in Tennessee. Kenny and Chris loved to clear land on my dad's tractor, and Gret was thrilled to spend the day riding horses on my aunt's farm. On hot summer days at my mom's house the kids could ride on a boat and play in the lake. After a few trips the kids knew every word to "American Pie" and many Paul Simon songs.

We decided to venture beyond visiting relatives and take a big trip to Branson, Missouri, where there were many family activities and something special for each of the kids. We bought tickets for magic shows and scouted out the best putt-putt golf courses.

On the plane, I became more and more distracted by growing stiffness and soreness in my back. I left my seat several times to stretch, and stood for a while in the back of the plane, bending and flexing my legs. By the time we landed I could hardly stay in my seat because of cramping. I was anxious to get off the plane, thinking maybe the angle of the seat or twisting to talk to the kids caused the problem.

I wiped sweat from my face and tried to remember if I took my morning medication in the chaos of getting everyone to the airport on time. Yes I did, with breakfast as usual. I swallowed hard, nauseated by vivid memories of my life under the dark cloud of uncontrolled pain.

Walking through the airport didn't relieve the cramping, and I struggled to manage our bags. I stopped to dump toothpaste and little shampoo bottles out of a Ziploc bag from our luggage, and filled the bag with ice at a soda station near the exit. We picked up our rental car, and I slipped the bag of ice behind my back to help calm the cramping.

When we made it to Branson we decided to walk around until we could check into our room later that afternoon. The kids had fun exploring the shops and assessing the attractions. My back began cramping so badly I was having trouble picking up my feet. I bought the kids some ice cream so we could sit down for a few minutes and I could rest my back. I found again that I couldn't sit, and paced as the kids enjoyed their treat.

After a few difficult hours following the kids around and trying very hard not to dampen their enthusiasm, we checked into our room. I stretched out on the bed with fresh ice under the small of my back while the kids unpacked and inspected the room. I took as much pain medication as I thought I safe, hoping that I would feel better soon and not ruin our vacation.

We had tickets to see Chinese acrobats and visited the gift shop while we waited for the theater to open. The kids were excited about toys they had never seen before. They played with Chinese yo-yos, and plates they could spin on a stick. The pain in my back was no better and was wearing on me. I was tired and quiet.

As we entered the theater, I looked at the fold-down seats with a sense of dread, but found that they were much more comfortable than I had expected. A few minutes after the show began, however, I couldn't find a comfortable position and became very restless because of a stabbing pain in the center of my lower back. I positioned my purse behind my back, and then under my thighs in an attempt to change the pressure on my back. Neither helped. I ended up standing in the back of the room, slowly bending and straightening my legs to try to relax my lower back. I watched the kids more than the acrobats, trying to make sure they were enjoying the show and not worrying about me.

The kids were exhausted after such a busy day and fell asleep as soon as we returned to our room. I was not so lucky. My back muscles were in knots, shooting pain down my legs and causing me to tense unnaturally and struggle to breathe. Ice helped relieve the cramping and reduce the pain, so I refilled the bag throughout the night. I was cold and the ice was uncomfortably lumpy, but I was able to get a little sleep.

I woke the next morning feeling the same. During putt-putt golf I just leaned on my club, trying not to throw up from pain and exhaustion as the kids played. As we finished the eighteenth hole and I stepped forward to return my club, my legs gave out without warning and I fell hard on my knees. I was shocked and embarrassed, and disturbed by the concerned look on the kids' faces.

"Wow, that was weird!" I stood and acted like it was no big deal.

I brushed dirt off my knees and walked ahead, but I was

shaken. Nothing like that had ever happened before. Did I fall because of my back, or was something wrong with my legs too? What was going on?

We picked up lunch and I took the kids to the pool at the motel. I thought they would have fun playing in the water, and I could relax my back. Swimming is good for a bad back, right?

The kids did have fun, but I made my back much worse. The constant movement of the water pushed and pulled my body, which caused my back to flex and twist more than usual. The pain and cramping were unbearable. I tried walking around outside the pool while the kids played, but I found no relief. I got everybody out of the pool and we went to our room to change. I then lay with my back on the floor, knees bent and feet up on a chair. It was the only position I could find that would give me any relief.

Chris watched television while Gret looked through tourist brochures we picked up when we checked in. Kenny sat outside the room in a plastic chair playing his Game Boy. The kids ate leftover sandwiches and snack crackers from a vending machine for dinner, then I talked them through getting ready for bed from the floor. They fell asleep with the television on as I lay on the carpet with tears sliding down my cheeks. I was hungry and tired and couldn't sleep.

I crawled to the bathroom, unable to walk. I stood and held myself up by grabbing the sides of the sink. My legs were weak and unstable.

I looked at myself in the mirror. What was I going to do? I couldn't go to the emergency room. What would I do with the kids?

Again my knees gave out and I almost smacked my chin on the sink. I took more pain medicine in desperation and paced around the room, slowly bending my knees and trying to loosen the muscles in my back. I finally fell asleep on the floor with my feet on the chair.

The next morning I woke to the sound of the television. Chris was up and had opened the curtains. Gretchen and Kenny stirred, complaining about the bright light. Chris eventually closed the curtains, and the kids lounged on the bed watching game shows.

My several hours on the floor helped relieve the cramped muscles, and I pulled my feet off the chair and waited for blood to return to my legs before attempting to stand. I was sore, but I felt better. I got the kids up and dressed, and we headed out for brunch.

We enjoyed a big meal of bacon and eggs, and sat around the restaurant table planning our day. We had dinner with a magic show in the evening, but nothing scheduled until then. Gret and Kenny wanted to go to the *Titanic* museum, but Chris did not. We decided to drive over later to see if we could change his mind.

As we slipped out of the booth, I realized that my back was again tightening up. It felt like I need to stretch, but any movement caused the muscles to catch and seize, taking my breath away. Sitting on a wooden bench for the entire meal had probably irritated it again.

We drove around a while and the kids spotted a strip of stores they wanted to explore. We parked the car, walked past jewelry and clothes shops, then the kids bounced into a shoe store, which surprised me. Why would they want to look at shoes?

Once inside, I saw the shelves of souvenirs that had captured the kids' attention. I passed racks of keychains and shot glasses, then stopped in front of a huge section of shoes with brands I didn't recognize. They looked comfortable and practical. I picked up a pair, opening and closing the Velcro strap. Maybe they were for older customers?

I turned to watch the kids as I leaned against a display, trying to take some pressure off my back. I slowly lifted one foot up and gently put it down, and then the other. Sweat began to stream down my face.

A young, energetic salesperson walked up and asked if I was okay.

"I'm fine," I said with frustration in my voice.

I told him I had chronic back problems and started to walk away to round up the kids, hoping my legs wouldn't give out and cause me to fall to the floor.

"I have the perfect thing for you!" he said. "Please follow me."

I hesitated, not really in the mood to try on shoes. He walked quickly to the rear of the building where tall sheets of unpainted wood created a wall, sectioning off a narrow space at the back of the store. He opened a door in the center and stepped inside. I slowly followed, wondering if I should just get the kids and leave.

In the back room, cardboard boxes were piled on the floor and pieces of shelving leaned against the wall. Clearly it was a storage area. But against the temporary wall, several narrow, wooden tables were lined up side by side a few feet apart. What was this place?

Gesturing toward the tables, the salesperson talked about how they had helped people with knee pain and hip pain, diabetes, and fibromyalgia. He said they improved cardiac health and helped people lose weight.

I stuck my head out of the doorway and motioned for the kids to join me. I didn't want them wandering off while I was distracted. Plus, I was beginning to plan a quick exit.

"Have a seat!" He stood at the head of the table closest to us.

Weird. Were they giving massages back there? He asked me to lay on the table. I looked at the kids and they nodded. I noticed a small white machine about the size of a toaster oven at the foot of the table, with something like a blue Frisbee on top. The man pulled a blue fabric cover over the blue disc and said that I should put my feet on it. I lay down and put my feet on it.

The salesman said the machine's vibrations would eliminate the pain in my back. I swung my legs over and quickly slid off the table. There was no way I was going to let anything further irritate my back. I could hardly walk as it was.

"It won't hurt you, it will only make you feel better!" he said. "You can stop it at any time if you don't like it."

I lay back down, questioning my judgment. What was I doing trusting this guy I just met in a shoe store to give me medical treatment?

I stared at the ceiling, holding my breath, and let him turn on the machine at the lowest setting.

"You have to start slowly at first," he explained. "After you get used to it you can use a higher setting for a longer time."

He set the timer for six minutes and left me alone. I think I fell asleep. When the timer sounded a loud "ping!" I climbed off the table and realized there was no cramping in my back. The shooting, stabbing pain was gone too. I took a couple of steps. No problem! The skin on my legs felt a little itchy from the vibrations, and the muscles in my back were sore from the earlier cramping, but I felt much better. What just happened??

It took more than the spending money I had planned for the entire trip, but I bought one of the machines. Several times a day for the rest of our vacation, we returned to the motel room so I could lay on the floor and vibrate my feet. I quickly moved beyond the recommended use to shorter intervals between expanded sessions needed to completely relax the muscles in my back.

I was able to sleep at night, sit through meals and entire shows with the kids, swim, play multiple rounds of putt-putt golf, and walk for hours. On the flight home I was washed with a sense of relief and tranquility as I watched the boys sleeping peacefully next to me.

I glanced down at the amazing little machine carefully tucked under the seat in front of me, and laughed out loud at the randomness and significance of walking into that bizarre shoe store.

Chapter Eight

ROLLER-COASTER RIDE

My back continued to spasm after we returned home from Branson. The kids went back to their normal routines, but I found myself suspended between my naturally playful, adventurous self and the cautious, reserved person I had become when I was trying to protect myself from pain.

Over the following weeks I used the vibrating machine more and more frequently, even throughout the night to loosen the twisted muscles in my back enough for me to sleep. Eventually it no longer helped even at the highest settings and I stored it in a closet.

I couldn't understand what had changed. I was taking the same amounts of anti-inflammatories and pain medications that were working beautifully before, but they were no longer having any effect. The pain and cramping were worse than ever. I was terrified to think that my respite was over and that I was going to return to a life firmly centered on pain.

Should I have known my relief was only temporary? I never thought about that possibility, but maybe I shouldn't have been surprised, since my back had progressively worsened for years. It seemed ridiculous, looking back, to think that somehow something was different and the problem just went away. Did I simply ignore a likely outcome that I didn't want to consider?

I returned, frustrated and confused, to my primary care doctor. He again referred me to a spine surgeon for an MRI. I returned to the same surgeon I'd seen before, hoping this time he would be able to help me. His reputation and reviews were stellar, and I really liked that he was an instructor and performed cutting-edge research. If anything could be done, he would know about it.

I was in the same exam room as before, poking the rubbery nerves sticking out of a little spine model, when the doctor came in with the disc from my new MRI. I watched as he scanned dozens of images on his computer screen until he found what he was looking for.

"These are your vertebrae, and this is your spinal cord," he said, tapping his finger on the big, dark, chunky blocks on the screen, then tracking the long, thick white line.

I knew this from earlier visits and the posters on every wall, but I didn't say anything.

"The discs in your lower back are more degenerated and compressed than before. Do you see here?" One by one he circled three areas near the bottom of the image. "This disc is herniated and these two are basically gone. These lower vertebrae are likely fusing together without the discs that should serve as cushions between them."

I could see that the top four vertebrae were separated by big, white spaces, which were apparently healthy disc like in the desktop model, but the lower vertebrae were pressed together with only dark lines between them.

"Surgery is only advised when a patient experiences numbness down the legs, indicating nerve compression in the lower back," he said.

"Sometimes I feel like my left leg could easily dislocate from my hip," I explained, wondering if I should lie about my symptoms. "And I do feel pain down into my legs from my back. But not numbness. My biggest complaint is the terrible pain and cramping in my back."

He studied me carefully, then opened a drawer and removed a rod almost a foot long. He held it up and said, "I don't recommend it, but rods can be implanted to stabilize your spine. There is about a sixty percent chance that surgery will result in a permanent inability to control your bladder."

As unhappy as I was with my situation, this did not sound like an ideal solution. We studied each other as I realized I was disappointed but not surprised, and saw that he was struggling as much as I was with the reality that I was suffering and he couldn't help me. The compassion in his eyes distracted me and kept me from sharing my frustration.

I left with another order for physical therapy, a referral to a pain specialist, and new prescriptions for pain medications and anti-inflammatories.

With great hesitation, I tried physical therapy again. Both my primary care doctor and spine surgeon were confident it would help, and they agreed on the best therapist in the area. Vowing to be open-minded and optimistic, I followed my therapist's exercise plan exactly and pushed myself during the sessions.

One afternoon in a typical therapy session I sat on a giant exercise ball with my feet flat on the ground, gently rolling to one side, then center, then the other side, then center. I'd learned to go only a little distance to the side to avoid triggering a spasm, but the movement still caused hot, stabbing pain. After completing three sets of ten, I moved to a giant padded table about two feet off the ground to continue my exercises. Another patient was on his side counting quietly as he lifted a hand weight a few inches off the mat and slid over to make room for me. On my back I pulled one knee to my chest, put the knee down, and then the other. My back suddenly cramped tightly, causing severe pain and difficulty moving my legs.

Sweating and shaking, I told my therapist that I was struggling and beginning to feel nauseous. She suggested a different exercise, and I moved to my hands and knees. She showed me how to raise one leg into the air behind me so that it was level with my back, then bring my knee into my chest. After two of these I raced to the bathroom to throw up.

When my stomach was empty I left the gym without a word to my therapist. I think she said something about trying some moist heat, but I ignored her. I was struggling to walk, and knew I couldn't talk. Finally, in my car, I tipped my seat back and passed out. It was the last time I went to therapy.

My visits to a pain specialist were much more effective.

I had no idea what to expect as I wrote my name on the sign-in sheet and took a seat in the waiting room. I felt out of place in my jeans and sweatshirt because the other patients, men and women, were in business suits. The room was shiny and modern, everything a classy blue/gray and silver. Could I afford this treatment? I thought I should have asked more questions about insurance and charges when I scheduled the appointment.

I filled out a stack of forms and took them with me when my name was called. A nice young man in blue scrubs took my clipboard and led me through a narrow hallway to a row of small changing rooms. He opened one of the doors and pointed out the gown hanging on the opposite wall and the floor-to-ceiling locker with a key in the lock. I stripped to my underwear and hung my clothes in the locker, put on the gown, took the key, and met him in the hallway.

He escorted me to a huge open room with a large X-ray machine and a wide treatment table in the center. The overhead lights were dimmed, but bright lamps lit workstations lining the walls. A tall, professional-looking man in a purple button-down shirt and tie pulled on his white coat as he rushed from a corner to greet me. The assistant introduced him as the doctor, then placed my paperwork on the big table and retreated into the glow of a nearby workstation.

"Hi!" the doctor said as he warmly shook my hand. "It's nice to meet you!"

I was cold in my socks and underwear with the back of my gown wide open, and a little self-conscious with the assistant behind me. I glanced around the room and wondered what was about to happen.

"I've reviewed your MRI and the report from your spine surgeon," he said, leaning into my line of vision to get my attention. "I'm sure I can help with your back pain. I can place some medicine into the affected areas of your back, which should give you significant relief."

"It can be a bit of a process," he said, picking up my papers and writing a short note on the top page before walking them over to his assistant. "Especially if your pain originates from multiple locations. First we need to pinpoint the exact areas to treat. Today I would like to inject a numbing medicine into the spot I think is likely causing you the most problems, then you go about your normal activities and see how you feel. If you experience relief, come back in a couple of weeks and I will inject a longer-acting anti-inflammatory into the same area. If you still have pain, we will identify another area to focus on. What do you think?"

I was in. I signed consent papers, accepting a very slight but serious risk of infection or paralysis. Nothing bad really happened, right? I was sure it was just a legal requirement and not something I actually needed to consider.

The assistant positioned me on the table, then rubbed disinfectant over my lower back. The doctor used the X-ray machine to guide a needle into my spine where he thought the treatment would be most effective.

On my belly with my cheek against the cold table, I was suddenly aware of every inch of my body. I could feel my bones pressing against the hard surface and desperately wanted to change position. The realization that there was nothing at all preventing me from movement almost caused me to panic. I clearly had a major role in my risk of injury. *Shouldn't I be strapped down?* There was a needle millimeters from my spinal cord. What if I sneezed?

My mind was racing but my body was completely still as my heart rate soared and I fought an overpowering need to jump off the table. The doctor, surely aware of my sudden silence and my muscles frozen in fear beneath his fingers, started to talk. He asked questions about my kids and shared stories about his own family, engaging me and helping me to relax. I have no idea how he maintained such lively conversation while he mastered such a delicate procedure. After about twenty minutes he was done, and the assistant placed a tiny Band-Aid on my back. I was on my way, excited about the prospects of this new treatment and encouraged by the warmth of my new physician.

Over the next six months the pain doctor was able to identify and successfully treat several areas in my back, giving me a much-needed break from pain. While I was not able to return to a completely carefree lifestyle, I was able to sleep at night and move through my day without experiencing breathtaking pain or spasms.

The company I worked for was regularly recognized as a high-performing organization and won a number of impressive awards. One of the successful business strategies was to teach all employees to continuously look for opportunities to do things better, and to create a team of full-time experts in problem solving and process improvement who would lead large-scale projects and train and mentor staff.

I was selected to become a full-time expert. At first I resisted, not interested in leaving my area of research for something that sounded to me like a business fad. But as I progressed in my training I realized the power of being able to analyze any process, and really enjoyed learning about other parts of the organization. The goals of my first projects included decreasing the number of biological samples stored incorrectly, reducing the cost of chemicals used in one of our laboratories, improving employee retention during their first year, and decreasing the time needed to orient new staff.

As I completed my first round of projects and immersed myself in my new role, the medication injected into my spine began to wear off. I was reminded of the complete control pain could have over my life. My exciting job and the kids barely entered my thoughts after several sleepless nights and with pain so severe I couldn't eat.

The injections provided relief for several weeks, but they could only be repeated every three months, which was not often enough to maintain their effectiveness. The couple of weeks before the next injection were miserable. After several cycles the treatments no longer worked at all. Fortunately there was another option. Following the same process as before, the doctor inserted the needle into my spine but instead of injecting medication he heated the needle to deaden the nerves in my back.

The new treatment was longer-lasting but not permanent. Feeling like I had a free pass with an expiration date, I decided to take the kids to Disney World. It's a trip they had asked about for years, but one that I had never been able to afford. With an unexpected bonus from work I made reservations at a Disney hotel, booked our flight, and bought park tickets.

Gretchen researched and planned our trip, strategically scheduling times to visit popular rides and booking a special dinner at each of the four parks. She and Kenny took advantage of extra park hours for Disney hotel guests, sometimes returning to our room long after Chris and I were asleep and leaving again early the next morning. They were teenagers, old enough to take the Disney bus to the parks without me. Chris and I were happy to spend the majority of the day with Gret and Kenny, then lounge in the pool or watch a little television before going to sleep.

While I didn't expect to have any issues with my back, stressful memories of our trip to Branson were constantly on my mind. Fear that I would ruin the vacation or that I wouldn't be able to take care of the kids haunted me even as the days passed without the hint of a problem.

I was cautious and joined the kids on the slow train through the park and on the tranquil jungle cruise, but happily held bags as they hopped on the more thrilling rides. Their description of a one-hundred-foot free fall on the Tower of Terror left me weak and shaken as I vividly imagined the pressure on my nonexistent discs when the ride abruptly stopped its forty-mile-an-hour descent just feet from slamming to the ground.

Toward the end of the trip, however, I was feeling confident enough to risk a roller-coaster ride with Kenny. The kids knew about my love of roller coasters and were on the lookout for one with minimal drops and thumps. Expedition Everest was the one. It was fast, but not too jarring by their standards. By this time the kids were almost as sensitive to activities that might irritate my back as I was.

Other than a slight hesitation out of habit as I delicately lowered myself onto the hard plastic seat, I wasn't really concerned.

The ride was fantastic! Fast and smooth. I didn't know anything about the attraction's story and laughed as we raced up a sharp incline through a mountain and faced what appeared to be a broken track at the top. We reversed direction, then entered a very dark cave. As we shot out of the darkness going backward at fifty miles per hour I looked over at Kenny to see if he was reacting to the loud, piercing scream that started as soon as the roller coaster raced away from the broken track. It wasn't until I saw him looking back with raised eyebrows and an open-mouthed laugh that I realized the scream was coming from me.

A few months after Disney I was struggling with my back again. I went through another round of nerve-deadening treatments with poor results. I was right back where I started before my first treatment.

Late one afternoon at work I was explaining the benefits of diagramming a process to a classroom full of business leaders when I froze. I put one leg forward to walk toward the front row of tables, and knew I would fall if I shifted my weight to that foot. All day my back had been cramping, and suddenly the muscles were clamped tight. The pain was unbearable. All eyes were on me as I stopped talking in midsentence. I completely lost my train of thought and tried desperately to figure out what to do. It was difficult to breathe.

I took a few shuffled baby steps and leaned forward with my palms pressed onto the smooth surface of the closest table, dripping sweat only inches from the concerned face of the person sitting across from me. Barely held upright by my shaking arms, I said without looking up, "Let's break here and pick up in the morning."

The group was surprised by the abrupt close and sat quietly for a second, then filed out of the room quickly when they realized they had a couple of hours of free time. I climbed onto the table and rolled onto my back with my knees bent. That's how one of my coworkers found me an hour later when he came to help me carry flip charts and handouts back to our office. He brought me some ice and after a while I was able to walk back to my desk, where I took an extra pain pill. I was unsure if taking an extra dose of the controlled substance was illegal and if I was putting myself at risk for harmful side effects, but I just wanted to be able to reduce the pain enough to go home.

That night I threw my pillow and blanket onto the floor, hoping the stable, flat surface would help reduce the spasms. Over the next several nights I slid a small folded towel under the small of my back to prevent sagging, and built up a stack of pillows beneath my knees.

I slept well on the floor, but woke up in the morning with my back so stiff I could hardly move. After experimenting with a wedge of couch cushions and pillows beneath my upper body, I found I felt much better in a partially inclined position. The problem was that I usually slid off the stack during the night, even when I pushed myself into the corner of my room.

I tried sleeping in a recliner, but no combination of pillows or rolled-up towels created a neutral position for my back. One night I fell asleep on the couch with my head propped up in the corner between the arm and the back cushion, and woke up in the same position the next morning without much pain or stiffness. With some fine tuning to perfectly place pillows in the gap between my elevated back and the cushions, the couch was exactly what I needed.

After a few months of monopolizing the living room at night, I moved the couch into my bedroom and leaned my mattresses against the wall. Eventually the couch became a permanent fixture in my room and I gave away my bed.

For my first major project at work I was asked to facilitate a weeklong session to integrate a newly acquired business into our organization. Leaders from our company and the new one would come together to identify and begin to address gaps and overlaps in business practices and services. In ninety days we needed to be working together as one, so the goal of our session was to agree on new common practices and create a detailed plan of the steps needed to get there.

I was terrified. Not because of the large number of high-level leaders I would need to engage and direct or the amount of work we needed to achieve in a short time, but because I was afraid my back would hurt so badly I wouldn't be able to walk or talk. I would have to travel to an unfamiliar business site, and stay in a hotel room without my customized sleeping arrangements. Nobody could step in for me if I ran into trouble.

I spent weeks planning large sessions and breakout groups, preparing the approach I would use to uncover everything that needed to be done without getting lost in the details.

I arrived for the meeting a day early to familiarize myself with the location, and to practice my opening presentation. It was Sunday, and the offices were closed. I paced back and forth in the huge ballroom-like space as I clicked through my slides, speaking with great conviction to rows of empty chairs until I no longer stumbled over my words.

At the hotel that evening I was critically analyzing the thick mattress topper on the bed when my boss called.

"Hi, Dee! Just wanted to see if you are ready. You know this merger is really important to our organization. It has to be fast, and seamless. We have no flexibility in the timeline and no room for error."

He sounded much more nervous than I was. I realized it must have been very difficult for him to be responsible for a key project when he had no control over the outcome.

"I'm ready," I told him. "I won't let you down."

I really wanted to do a good job, not only to please my boss but also to help the two businesses come together in a way that would be effective and efficient. Plus, I really enjoyed working on large-scale projects and would be given more opportunities in our big company if I was successful.

After dinner in my room at the hotel and a few more practice runs through my material, I was ready to go to sleep. The bed was much too soft to offer any support, so I decided to give the boxy couch a try. It was pale green with rough fabric and firm cushions. I spent half an hour placing and adjusting pillows against the arm and back to eliminate gaps as much as possible. I needed my spine to be completely neutral to avoid irritation or spasms.

I put my head on the hard wooden arm of the couch and fell asleep, hoping to wake up for any twitch or ache so I could adjust my position.

I woke the next morning refreshed and energized. I bent and stretched my legs to test for sensitivity, but there was none. In the shower I was ready to let the hot water warm any tight muscles in my back, but it was not necessary. Wow! Okay, so far so good! I tried not to think about how badly the night could have gone and how quickly issues with my back could ruin all my plans, and left for the meeting.

All morning I was on my feet in front of the large group, then spent the afternoon bouncing between smaller conference rooms to check on the progress of each team. By the end of the day I was exhausted but very happy. The group was working well together and both organizations were beginning to appreciate the experience and expertise of their new peers. The tone was set and we were right on schedule.

In my hotel room that first night I dropped my work bag onto the bed and skipped around the small room with my arms above my head, repeating *"Yes, yes!"* I did it! All day long I was able to focus without thinking about my back. There were no embarrassing disasters. I pushed on the muscles on each side of my spine above my belt. A little tender, but nothing like the sickening pain I usually felt by the end of the day. I shook my head and laughed. Wow. What a relief. I didn't understand what was going on, but I was very, very appreciative.

By Wednesday afternoon I was no longer thinking about my back at all and was totally engaged in our efforts. The teams had transitioned from learning the details of each other's processes to designing new and improved ones. Clearly motivated by action, the leaders were driven and energized.

On Friday afternoon we held a closing meeting to present the new processes and action plans to senior leaders from both organizations. My boss and several others attended in person, while more joined remotely. Each team spoke about their designs with pride and confidence. It was clear that everyone was working well together and that the businesses would be successfully integrated by the deadline. I was especially pleased that everyone was engaged and ready to move forward.

We all happily accepted congratulations and thanks from our bosses. We were excited about all that we accomplished but were finally feeling the toll of such a grueling week. The big room seemed unusually quiet and still as the last attendees packed up to go home.

Chapter Nine

ACCOMMODATIONS

My reprieve ended abruptly on Saturday morning when I stood up from the couch in my bedroom and immediately crashed to the floor. My back muscles were clenched and my legs wouldn't hold my weight. I rolled onto my back and slid my legs onto the couch to try to calm the spasms and my suddenly racing mind.

What was going on? How could I feel great for an entire week, then suddenly be unable to stand? I was *SO* grateful it hadn't happened the week before.

I thought it must have been my couch. I felt fine and supported when I fell asleep, but something clearly was different. Maybe the cushions were too soft or the pillows moved beneath me when I slept.

Over the next few weeks I experimented with different positions, pillows, and cushions on the couch. I even slid a piece of plywood under the cushions in case the couch itself was saggy. Nothing helped, and I gave up on standing when I first woke up. Instead I would slowly roll off the low couch, very careful to move my upper and lower body together to avoid the slightest twist, and crawl around my bedroom. The movement was painful, but loosened my back enough so I could stand within a couple of minutes.

It wasn't unusual for me to wake up several times during the night to slightly adjust my position. Keeping my spine perfectly straight when I slept was very unnatural for me, but absolutely necessary to avoid days of debilitating pain and cramping.

One night, barely awake, I realized I was leaning toward the outside of the couch. I rolled my head back to the center, then pushed my hands down beside my hips to lift and slide a little closer to the back of the couch. I immediately sat straight up with a shocking bolt of pain through my lower back.

I usually bent my knees and pushed my heels down as I carefully lifted myself, but this time my legs were motionless. My lower body stayed still while my upper body moved, causing a sudden bend at my waist and excruciating pain. I tried again, and realized my legs were frozen. Moving them was not difficult or painful, it was impossible. They wouldn't budge.

I sat perfectly still, petrified. *No, no, no, no. Please don't let me be paralyzed. Am I paralyzed?!*

I reached down and picked up one leg, pulling my knee to my chest and ignoring the blazing pain in my spine. I could feel my touch on my skin, unlike the detached sandbag feeling of my arm when I woke up with it under me. Maybe that was a good sign? *Come on, come on!* I pulled my leg up and put it back down until I could move it on its own. I threw my head back and blew out my breath. Wow.

My nocturnal paralysis became a common event but didn't seem to have any residual effect during the day. I became so sensitive to movement at night I wedged pillows all around my body to try to keep myself still, but often stirred a little and woke up in horrible pain. I would then lie awake for hours in tears from exhaustion and frustration, afraid to fall asleep again.

No number of pills helped the situation. Out of desperation one night after staring at the ceiling in my bedroom for hours, I dragged myself to the kitchen for a bottle of wine. I was angry and desperate, tired of the pain and the constant fog from lack of sleep. Wine always made me sleepy and I thought maybe it would provide a much-needed solution.

I found a corkscrew and opened the bottle in the moonlight from a small kitchen window. I drank half the bottle without a glass and without pausing for breath, pushed the cork back in, and went back to my room where I passed out on the couch.

Wine did allow me to sleep soundly for a few hours without any movement. I considered remotely whether drinking alcohol with consistent use of prescription pain pills was a good idea, but I didn't care. I had to sleep. I bought a dozen bottles of wine with twist-off tops and stored them in my bedroom closet. I always kept one by my bed so I didn't have to go far when I needed it.

The problem with drinking alcohol was that I woke up several hours later extremely restless and unable to go back to sleep. Depending on how miserable I was at bedtime, sometimes it was worth it. I was getting only about four hours of sleep each night if I was lucky, and began carrying caffeine pills in my pocket to nibble off chunks during the day to help me stay awake. I couldn't drink enough coffee to be effective.

The severity of my pain and cramping continued to escalate. My pain was most intense when I stood still and the cramping worse when I moved, so my discomfort was always peaked. I discovered disposable adhesive heat pads, little miracles that calmed the muscles and helped me feel a little better. In no time I was using them constantly, often with two or three lined up at my waist to cover my entire lower back.

Even with heat and prescription drugs I was often unable to walk or speak because of pain and cramping. I could no longer downplay my situation. At work when our process improvement team planned training sessions I signed up for support rather than teaching roles so the class wouldn't be affected if I was out of commission. I turned down opportunities to travel for large-scale projects, requesting instead to manage smaller, local projects that allowed flexibility in my schedule and in my interactions with other people.

I left work early one Wednesday afternoon in so much pain I simply drove to my doctor's office without an appointment. He gave me refills for pain pills and anti-inflammatories, and a new prescription for muscle relaxants. He said the new medicine wasn't for regular use because it would likely make me very sleepy, but should provide some relief from my most severe symptoms. That sounded wonderful. I didn't need to function, I just needed a break from the pain.

I filled the prescription immediately. Once home, I walked through the house to the kitchen for a glass of water to take one of the new pills. I dropped my purse and keys on the table between Kenny and Chris, who mumbled hello without looking up from their mounds of homework.

From her room above the driveway, Gretchen heard me come in. She bounced down the stairs and ran to the kitchen, skillfully slid in her socks to a stop next to me, and wrapped me in a bear hug.

I stiffened, trying to protect my back. I put my hand on her shoulder and gave a small squeeze in a feeble attempt to assure her that I wasn't rejecting her affection. She didn't notice.

"Hey Mom, can we drive? It's early so we can go for a couple of hours!"

Gret wanted to spend every possible minute in the car. She'd earned her learner's permit and was required to log forty hours behind the wheel with an adult passenger before she could get her license. A major step toward her innate goal of maximum independence was within reach.

I stared at her with the prescription bottle in my hand and a big lump in my throat. There was no way I could sit in a car. I barely made it home.

I filled a glass with water and leaned against the counter for support as I popped a pill in my mouth. I wanted to say yes, to watch Gret's face light up as I told her we could drive until dark, maybe picking up food while we were out and making a delivery to the boys. I wanted to hear about her day and her plans for the weekend, about the car she wanted to buy and the jobs she would get to pay for it. I wanted to be part of this milestone event with my oldest child, wanted this sense of normalcy.

Instead, I walked past the kitchen table into the open living room and pulled a blanket off the back of the couch. "I can't, Gret. I'm really sorry." I lowered myself to the floor and put my legs on the coffee table. "My back is killing me."

She looked at my pale, strained face, then my dirty shoes on the table.

"Are you okay?"

Her thrill over my early arrival was long gone. She glanced at the boys, who looked up when they heard the concern in her voice. I saw their worried expressions and held back tears. My life was wrecked enough; I didn't want the kids to be affected too.

"I'll be fine," I said, with my eyes closed to shut out their faces. "Can your dad ride with you?"

With a little too much enthusiasm to be credible, she said, "Oh, sure, that would be great! I'd like to get more experience driving his car anyway!"

Gret gently pulled off my shoes and placed them under the table, then put a pillow under my head and another blanket over my feet. She told the boys they needed to find dinner for themselves.

I fell asleep on the floor. When I woke up hours later the house was dark and quiet.

At the advice of my doctor, I tried a small, portable nerve stimulator attached to my back. It helped for a short time but quickly became ineffective. I added pain pills to the caffeine in my pocket and found myself increasing the frequency I took them to get through the day.

After months with no change in my situation I noticed one day at work that I was not struggling to breathe when I walked. The cramping was much less than usual, and the pain was dull rather than stabbing. *What was going on?*

The only thing that was different was the shoes. The shoes! I was wearing the ones I'd worn when my back felt great during the big integration event I facilitated at work. I'd known I would be on my feet all day for an entire week, so I wore shoes with a wide, thick rubber heel rather than the narrow, wobbly ones or wafer-thin flats I usually wore. The instability and lack of support of my regular shoes must have been further irritating my back.

Finally, something I could do to feel better! I threw all of my other shoes to the back of my closet and wore the very practical, clunky black leather shoes every day. After enjoying several weeks of reduced symptoms, I was confident enough in my improved health to accept an invitation to facilitate an off-site meeting with our local senior leadership team to set goals for the following year. It would be fun to help them brainstorm and vet projects, and I was looking forward to the challenge of keeping the group focused and helping to produce a strong plan by the end of the day.

I didn't notice my back getting tight and my legs getting shaky until late in the afternoon, when I turned around to write first-quarter volume goals on a flip chart. When my weight shifted my feet didn't move. I pitched forward and dropped to my hands and knees. With my head down I didn't see the reaction of the group, but I did hear their gasps. I crawled a couple of feet and managed to push myself up, then handed the marker off to one of the attendees sitting by the door as I dragged my concrete legs out of the room. I didn't make eye contact. I didn't want help, and I didn't want to talk. I felt humiliated and defeated. What I really wanted to do was hurl the marker into the wall.

I drove home and climbed into a tub of hot water. The heat was soothing and the water suspended me enough to take pressure off my back. As I regularly reheated the water throughout the evening, I wondered if the kids were okay. They were perfectly capable of taking care of themselves, but I felt guilty for not saying a word to them when I came home from work. I told myself they would knock on the door if they needed me, then slid deeper into the water.

Once fully relaxed, I tipped my head back and let the cold porcelain chill the skin on the back of my neck. It was nice to feel a sensation other than pain. I closed my eyes and wondered what I was going to do. This was no way to live. I woke up to freezing cold water several hours later, took a muscle relaxer, and went to sleep on the couch.

Convinced my shoes were a critical element for reducing pain, I was determined to find ones that would improve my situation. I knew I couldn't wear anything with a heel and that the shoes needed to be very wide. I'd always had wide feet, but in the past had no trouble squeezing them into any kind of shoe. Now my back was supersensitive to the alignment of my legs, which seemed to be affected by pressure on my feet.

I visited a huge number of shoe stores and tried dozens of pairs of shoes. Every one caused muscle spasms, back pain, and weakness in my legs within minutes of putting them on. Frustrated by the rarity of wide women's shoes, I broadened my search to include men's shoes that could possibly pass as professional-looking women's shoes, since a standard-width men's shoe was the same as a wide-width women's shoe.

During a determined visit to a huge shoe warehouse, I planted myself between the men's and women's selections for maximum variety. A kind sales woman came to my rescue when she noticed that I had discarded a large pile of cute women's shoes and was pulling on a heavy pair of men's wingtips with a look of desperation and disappointment. She asked a few questions and told me that I needed to replace the shoe insoles with something designed for my needs. She brought a variety of products for me to consider.

After much trial and error I finally found a pair of men's Adidas running shoes that I could comfortably wear if I replaced the insole with a hard plastic arch support sandwiched between two cushiony inserts. The shoes were extra wide and two sizes too big, and I switched the shoestrings for long bootlaces loosely tied so all the inserts and my feet would fit inside. A perfect balance of cushion and support, the shoes helped calm my irritated back.

I wore the black Adidas everywhere, regardless of the occasion. I colored the white stripes with a black Sharpie so they were less obviously athletic shoes, and at work I wore black or dark gray slacks with wide legs so the shoes would be less noticeable. While I was a little self-conscious about the impression they made, the shoes became my most precious possessions. They enabled me to function.

Kenny took band class in middle school and fell in love with the saxophone. I loved to hear him play as his skills developed, and even enjoyed his endless repetition of scales because of his incredible tone. When he played the music of his heroes Sonny Rollins or Charlie Parker, I would swear I was in a smoky bar in the 1950s. I had no idea how such a powerful and soulful sound came from such a slim-framed young man.

By high school Kenny was an award-winning musician and regularly played in concerts and competitions. I missed many performances because I was unable to travel and unable to sit in the audience. But when he was chosen from a highly competitive group of musicians to play in a statewide honor band with a renowned guest conductor, I was determined to attend.

I struggled and squirmed in a makeshift bed in the backseat of Phil's car as he drove three and a half hours to the concert hall in a gorgeous 250-year-old resort in the Allegheny Mountains. As I walked the halls of the historic hotel in my prized Adidas, the tightness in my back from the long ride loosened with every step. I felt a little underdressed in my wrinkled slacks and blouse, and drew a few stares from women in beautiful dresses and sharp suits.

Maybe they noticed me because I was clearly the happiest person in the building and not because the lighting made the stripes on my shoes glow purple.

I was ecstatic to be there. I wasn't slugging wine in a bathtub or supine on the living room floor, I was 200 miles from home supporting my son.

Kenny arrived for rehearsals two days earlier and I hadn't talked to him since he left home. Phil and I slipped into the performance hall, hoping for a minute to say hello, as the concert band vacated the stage and the jazz band began setting up. Kenny was adjusting his music stand when I waved my hand to get his attention. His eyes widened when he saw me, a big grin brightening his face. I was so happy at that moment I thought I would pop. Kenny clearly didn't expect to see me, and was probably relieved that I was well enough to be there as much as pleased that I would see his performance.

I sat with Phil for the first song, then quickly moved to the back of the long room when my back began to cramp. In the dim light fifteen feet behind the last row of chairs I could pace without notice, feeling stronger and energized. The only weakness I felt was when Kenny stood for a solo, with every one of the hundreds of people in the audience watching in anticipation. He mastered the piece like a pro, then blushed under thunderous applause as he returned to his seat and I started to breathe again.

Soon I needed the support my shoes provided all the time and could no longer go barefoot, even for the few minutes needed for a shower. I tried standing on a gardener's kneeling pad, a bath pillow, a folded-up towel, and shoe inserts, but none provided the support I needed. I replaced my showers with baths and looked for a pair of flip-flops.

After an exhaustive search, I found a pair of flip-flops I could stand on for about ten minutes before my back began to spasm. These were not $5 convenience store flip-flops, but rather $125 flip-flops with a built-in support device, which I found in a specialty shoe store at the mall during a mission to try every pair of flip-flops I saw until I found a pair that would work. Interestingly, they were one of the brands I noticed during our trip to Branson that I thought must have been designed for older customers. They were perfect. They were comfortable, and even had a felt foot bed so my feet wouldn't slide around when wet. They became my second most valued possessions after the Adidas.

As I concluded my efforts to find the right shoes, I started trying to address my difficulty sitting. I knew the pressure to my back from the seats I was using was adding to my discomfort, so I was anxious to find something different. I went to every office supply and furniture store I could find and tried every chair in every store. In addition to a number of ergonomic office chairs, one by one I bought a yoga ball chair, several lawn chairs and bar stools, a bicycle seat stool, and a kneeling chair.

Eventually nothing worked and I stopped sitting. I stood at the island in my kitchen for dinner while the kids ate at the table, and paced behind the couch when we watched television together. At work I created a stand-up desk by stacking several books and computer monitor risers, and stood in the back of the room during meetings.

Chapter Ten

DECLINE

While I was absorbed with accommodating my fragile back, I began to experience pain in other parts of my body. One morning my fingers hurt so badly I couldn't squeeze toothpaste out of the tube. Then, a few days later, I noticed a deep, stabbing pain in the bottom of my feet and a pins- and-needles sensation in the arch with every step. My left hip and the right ankle that I injured playing softball in high school started to ache constantly. The next week the joints of the big toe on my left foot became so sore I was unable to push it against the floor when I walked. Then my wrists hurt and burned when I moved them, and I developed very painful bunions on the outside of both big toes. My knees popped and made grinding sounds with any movement.

I had no idea what was going on. In the span of a couple of months pain consumed my entire body. Countless doctor visits resulted in similar orders to avoid the use of a specific body part, seek physical therapy, increase medications, or consider surgery.

I had surgery on one knee, and then the other. As I recovered from the second surgery and thought about whether my wrists or toes were the next highest priority, my skin began to change. Huge dry patches covered my ribs on both sides of my body, the skin between my toes split open, and my feet and hands became dry and scaly. My fingernails and fingertips cracked and peeled, and the skin on my knuckles split into deep cuts that became infected. I had canker sores in my mouth constantly, up to a dozen at one time, and acne on my face. I tried over-the- counter and prescription topical and oral medications, but abandoned them as they were minimally effective.

One beautiful spring morning I drove right past the building where I worked. A few miles later, when I realized what I'd done, I pulled into a gas station and parked the car. It wasn't the first time lately I'd driven past my intended destination, but this time I didn't just laugh it off and turn around. This time I was worried.

In the past week I'd forgotten to rinse the shampoo out of my hair before getting out of the shower, and left the gas burner on for hours after I finished using the stove. I'd become so forgetful I started writing notes to remind me about routine tasks such as moving the clothes from the washer to the dryer and checking the mail.

I knew something was wrong. No doubt all my medical issues were distracting, but I wasn't absorbed in thought or sidetracked by competing priorities. My mind was thick and slow. I wasn't thinking about anything.

After about fifteen minutes of sitting motionless while rushed commuters buzzed around me, I started the car and drove back to work. At my desk I opened my calendar and looked at the one-hour blocs with no coherent thought. Normally the entry "project review meeting" would prompt me to analyze data and prepare a presentation. I couldn't recall if I had done anything to prepare for that meeting at noon, or even which projects would be reviewed.

I was beginning to panic. I knew there were things I needed to be doing, but I had no idea what they were. I read my "to do" list several times, but the words didn't translate into meaningful information. I looked remotely around my desk for clues, then opened and closed my desk drawers. Nothing. Not even a spark of an idea. Finally I sent a message to our team saying that I wasn't feeling well, and went home.

At home I called my primary care doctor and scheduled an appointment for the next day. I had been handling every physical ailment as it arose, seeking treatment from the appropriate specialist for each specific problem. But with so many issues affecting so much of my body at once and my new inability to focus, I felt like I needed to tell one doctor everything that was going on.

In the lobby of the doctor's office the next morning, I signed in using a new computer system where I scanned my driver's license and swiped my credit card without bothering the busy receptionists. Before I could move across the room to wait, a nurse called my name and led me to an exam room I'd been in many times before. She took my blood pressure and said the doctor would be right in.

The doctor walked in as the nurse was walking out. He glanced at me as he placed his laptop on the small desk, then sat on the rolling stool. He seemed more serious than normal. He offered no smile and no greeting. I described all my symptoms and shared my concerns as he typed on the computer, then waited for him to look up. I wondered if he noticed the quiver in my voice. I knew something was terribly wrong, and was afraid to hear what he had to say. Did he already have a diagnosis based on what I told him? Would he tell me directly, or would I have to wait for confirmation from a specialist?

He listened to my heart and felt the glands in my neck, then declared, "You are under too much stress. Women your age work too hard and don't get enough rest."

I blinked, trying to direct my thoughts to the path he was taking. By the time I realized what he meant, he had returned to his computer. I studied the back of his head as the information soaked in. My shoulders dropped and my heart sank. I wanted to disappear.

Was I doing this to myself?!

I was embarrassed and ashamed. Of course, being a single mom with a full-time job and three active children kept me busy, but were they making me sick? I definitely *was* stressed about my health and my inability to do the things I wanted to do, but was I stressed by my life?

My health had become progressively worse as the kids grew older and more involved in activities outside the house, and money definitely was a concern, since older kids needed cars, insurance, and college tuition. Was I more worried than normal about something happening to them or about being able to take care of them?

I dragged my feet and hung my head, not wanting to make eye contact with anyone as I left the doctor's office. I felt that everyone knew I was unhinged and was laughing at me about it.

The doctor visit made me realize I was under a lot of stress. For a few weeks after the appointment I tried to be aware of any stressful thoughts or feelings and consider whether worry seemed to impact how I felt. I didn't really think so, and couldn't shake the sinking feeling that something was very wrong with my body. But my doctor didn't seem at all concerned about my physical health. He didn't even run any tests! There was no referral or follow-up visit to see how I was doing later. Was I exaggerating my symptoms? Should I see a therapist? I didn't really know what to do next or who could help me figure out what was going on.

I scheduled an appointment with a psychiatrist, partly to find out if I was making myself sick and partly because I wanted to talk more about my struggle to concentrate. I was afraid if I didn't take some action I was going to lose my job. That certainly would cause plenty of stress!

I wrote my name on a clipboard outside a sliding glass window between the small, bright waiting room and the unattended receptionist desk. I was the only one waiting and flipped through a couple of magazines until the doctor walked out with another patient and greeted me warmly. She was in her midfifties with shoulder-length brown hair, matching silver beaded earrings and necklace, and glasses perched on the tip of her nose. She wore a dark wool suit and low heels. She led me past several closed doors to her open office at the end of the hall. It was large, with two walls of windows overlooking a parking lot on one side and a small pond and gazebo on the other.

She placed a file on her large executive desk just inside the door and picked up a notepad, then walked to a living room-type area with a beautiful red and gold rug beneath a delicate coffee table in the center of the room. She offered an overstuffed chair or couch to me, and I chose one end of the couch. She sat with perfect posture in a high-back chair across from me.

The doctor watched me closely and listened carefully as I answered questions about my work and family situation. We talked about my medical history and where I felt I was struggling with my health. By the end of the session she told me she did not find my health challenges to be psychologically based, but provided a diagnosis of attention deficit disorder and a prescription for medication to help me focus.

Wow, okay. The knowledge that my physical issues were not created in my head was somehow comforting, but also unsettling because I still had no idea what was going on with my body.

Initially the ADD medication gave me energy and cleared my fogginess, but as my pain became even more severe my mind seemed to cloud up again too. I continued to take the medication even as it became much less effective because I was hopelessly confused without it.

In addition to the long-lasting ADD medicine I took twice daily, the psychiatrist prescribed a short-acting "as needed" treatment that I added to my drug pocket with caffeine and pain pills.

Suddenly I began having terrible pain in my neck, worse than in any other part of my body. The muscles in my neck were tight, pulling my shoulders up toward my ears in a constant shrug. The left side of my back became completely numb, but a sharp, burning pain radiated through my arms. I had to constantly shake my hands to try to rid them of cold and tingling, and regularly dropped whatever I was carrying because of reduced sensitivity in my fingers.

During a visit to the grocery, I felt strong electrical shocks in the palms of both hands as I pushed the cart through the store. I searched the cart for devices or cameras, sure that an electric current was somehow flowing through the cart or that someone was playing a joke on me. A few weeks later I felt this sensation in my hands every time I put them under a stream of water from the faucet, and realized it must have been caused by the irritated nerves in my neck.

I tried very hard to keep my hands apart, my elbows at my sides, and my head completely straight to avoid irritating my neck. Regardless of my diligence, every day by late afternoon I developed a blinding headache and nausea that lasted through the night. The only help I found was from a traction device I created one evening by dropping a rope over a doorknob and suspending a dish towel like a hammock to support my head as I stretched out on the floor. It really helped to lessen the tension in my neck, and I spent hours in this position staring at the ceiling as I listened to the kids' conversations and television shows in the next room.

Another appointment with my spine surgeon led to another MRI and another diagnosis of degenerated and compressed discs. But unlike my back, the discs in my neck could be fixed. Surgery could be performed to remove the degenerated discs and to screw a plate into the vertebrae that would limit movement and prevent pressure on the nerves. Little cylinders containing crushed-up cadaver bone would be inserted between the vertebrae to help the bones in my neck fuse together for permanent stabilization. Two of my discs were badly degenerated and would be removed, so the three vertebrae surrounding them would be fused together.

I didn't know that crushedup bone helped other bones fuse, or that cadavers were bone donors. Weird, and cool! The doctor assured me that the donor bones were completely sterilized so my body wouldn't reject them and they wouldn't make me sick. Of course I told the kids that the donor was probably a monster who would control my actions after surgery. They were all teenagers by then and just rolled their eyes at me.

The procedure went well and from the moment I woke up in my hospital room I felt like a new person. My headache and the tightness in my shoulders were gone. I no longer had pain in my arms and I could feel my fingers. Woohoo! The strong painkilling drugs were no doubt helping my overall sense of well-being, as I felt no pain in my back or any other areas of my body.

I was discharged from the hospital the next day with a more powerful pain medication than I was used to taking and instructions that told me what to expect over the following few days. The information very clearly stated that the surgical approach through the front of my neck would cause significant swelling and difficulty swallowing. I found that to be true and was unable to eat any food.

By the second day at home my throat shifted visibly to one side when I tried to drink small amounts of liquid until I eventually couldn't swallow anything, including my pain medication. Then, to my surprise, the swelling greatly reduced within a couple of hours. I thought an allergic reaction to the medication must have caused the extreme swelling. No problem; I just stopped taking it.

By the third day I wasn't able to eat anything solid, but could easily drink liquids. Even without the pain medication I felt fantastic. Nothing hurt. I slept on a recliner to keep my neck in a comfortable position, but I had no pain, even in my back.

I was shocked by this unexpected result. I called the surgeon to ask what he had done that would eliminate all of my pain for such a long time. Did it have something to do with manipulation of my spinal cord? Some kind of long-lasting nerve block?

The surgeon said he had done absolutely nothing that would affect any other part of my body and that I must be enjoying the effects of the pain medication. But I hadn't taken any pain medication for more than twenty-four hours. Was it so strong it could it last for more than a day and cause my body to respond so completely?

I hadn't experienced a complete lack of pain in many years. It was an amazingly liberating feeling, like an untethered balloon drifting in a gentle breeze.

With a soft brace on my neck and some residual queasiness from the anesthesia, I was unable to run a marathon like I thought I might be able to do with my newfound freedom. Instead, I piled on the couch with the kids for an entire day of movie watching. It had been years since I had even sat on a couch to watch television, much less mashed together at odd angles with three big people.

The next day the swelling in my throat had decreased enough for me to eat, and my pain returned to its normal intolerable state.

Chapter Eleven

COMING UNDONE

After my brief relief from pain after neck surgery, I was keenly aware of how much every joint in my body hurt. I felt like a zombie, mindlessly propelling my stiff and deteriorating frame through whatever I needed to do to get through the day.

Throughout that very cold winter, I was unable to get warm. I wore a coat all day at work with hand warmers dropped into the pockets to generate extra heat. After work I rushed home, shivering, to plunge my feet into a tub of hot water. Once warm enough to stop shaking I pulled on layers of clothes, a scarf, and a stocking cap. I didn't take anything off when I went to bed, just added more socks and crawled under a stack of blankets. I kept the heat turned up so high the kids wore shorts and T-shirts inside the house.

I didn't warm up with the weather, and by summertime I experienced a deeply concerning loss of color and feeling in my fingers and toes. Without warning, one or two of my fingers or toes would turn an absolute dead white for up to an hour at a time. They seemed to be influenced by something beyond my control because no amount of warming or shaking brought back the color or the feeling.

One hot Saturday morning at the grocery store, while snuggled in my sweatshirt and down vest, I began to feel very light-headed and became drenched in sweat. Suddenly exhausted, I just wanted to lay on the floor and rest. I crumpled against a display at the end of an aisle, so sleepy I couldn't move. I wasn't scared or embarrassed, just incredibly drained. After a few minutes I was okay and able to continue shopping.

I experienced similar episodes over the following few months. Research led me to believe this might have been a blood sugar problem, but after several rounds of testing my doctor ruled out diabetes. There clearly was a connection to food, however, since I could recover more quickly if I had something to eat. I learned to notice earlier warning signs and carried a granola bar with me everywhere I went.

As I was dealing with my inability to control my pain, to focus, to avoid skin infections, and to manage my body temperature, the horrible pain in my neck returned. I barely had the strength to support my head, and this time I had a horrible stabbing pain in my right shoulder. I felt like someone was twisting a knife in my upper arm. The only relief I found was from carrying a ten-pound weight in my right hand to drop my shoulder into a less excruciatingly painful position. My previous neck problems did not create any difficultly driving, but with this second round I was unable to hold my arms up while steering and unable to turn the key to start the car.

A fresh MRI of my neck showed another degenerated disc and an incomplete fusion of one of the disc spaces that had been surgically repaired. In addition, one of the screws holding the implanted plate in place was backing out of my vertebrae, which is apparently pretty unusual because they are locked during surgery. My surgeon was very surprised and disturbed by the dislodged screw, and insisted on showing me his surgical notes to prove that they were all secured before closing the wound.

My intense shoulder pain complicated the diagnosis and significantly lowered my spine surgeon's confidence in his treatment plan. He first wanted to investigate the shoulder issues.

He ordered another MRI to evaluate the condition of my shoulder. Preparation involved injecting dye into the joint, using a live X-ray for guidance. I was very familiar with this procedure because of my many visits to the pain clinic, where a live X-ray was used to place pain medication or introduce an electric current to a very specific position in my spine. The process was long and tedious, and I found it difficult to tolerate the trial and error as the doctor slowly manipulated the needle into place.

Because of my unease with going through the process again, I was excited and a bit punchy when I arrived at the radiology center. A very quiet young female technician led me to the procedure room, positioned me on the table beneath the X-ray machine, then quite formally introduced a middle-aged male doctor as he entered the room. He very slightly nodded his head in my direction, moved a stool a fraction of an inch, sat next to me, then without a word repositioned my shoulder.

In a desperate attempt to ease the tension and reduce my anxiety, I said, "If you were any good you could place the dye without an X-ray."

I regretted the words the second they tumbled from my mouth. The look of near panic on the technician's face horrified me. Everyone froze.

What was I thinking?!

The doctor's hand suddenly dropped from my shoulder. He stood and pushed the X-ray machine away. He looked down at me as a huge grin spread across his face.

"Would you like me to turn it off?" he asked.

I let out the breath I didn't realize I was holding. "Maybe for the next patient," I said.

After that the doctor and the technician were both very relaxed and personable, and the experience as pleasant as could be.

An orthopedic surgeon operated on my shoulder to address

degenerative changes, then four months later the spine surgeon performed the second surgery on my neck. After treatment for a postoperative infection and a frozen shoulder, the pain in my neck and shoulder was resolved. My challenge then, in addition to escalating cognitive and physical issues throughout my body, was total exhaustion.

I began to experience such a complete lack of energy I could barely function. I had been managing my symptoms to the best of my ability, but the exhaustion broke me.

I stood in the kitchen one morning, struggling to stay upright while drinking a cup of coffee. Kenny and Chris buzzed around me as they ate breakfast and prepared for school. I put my cup down on the kitchen island into a small circle of milk and immediately flushed with anger.

"Can't you clean up after yourselves?!" I snapped as I reached for a paper towel to wipe up the milk.

"I'm sorry, Mom," Kenny said as he looked at me sideways, surprised and concerned by my reaction. "I must've missed that spot."

"Can you guys clean this place up?!" I barked, waving my arm to broadly indicate the rest of the house. I hadn't been able to clean in weeks, and the dust on the furniture and dirty footprints on the kitchen floor served as constant reminders of my inability to manage my life. The boys would have gladly cleaned or helped with anything else I needed, but I didn't have the strength to ask. An emotional reaction in the moment was all I could do.

At work I stood at my desk truly feeling like I was going to collapse. Or maybe just melt into a puddle, like the Wicked Witch of the West. I desperately needed to sleep, so I booked a conference room for a couple of hours. This was a new practice I'd started a few weeks earlier in an attempt to put in a full day at work. In the conference room I was restless and angry, unable to get comfortable on the table or a chair. No matter how much pain I was in I always fell asleep within seconds of turning off the overhead light. For some reason this day was different.

I walked back to my desk and picked up the keys to my car. In the parking lot I climbed into the backseat and stretched out on my back. I didn't have the energy to drive home and didn't care if anyone walked by and saw me. I was so far from my normal life none of it seemed to matter. As I lay there, I thought of myself as a sea creature washed to shore, struggling to breathe as others passed by in a world very different from mine.

The bright sun overhead made my closed eyelids look red. With my knees bent and my hands neatly folded on my stomach, I performed a self-assessment. At forty-eight years old I wore shoes in the shower and couldn't sit. I walked without flexing my ankles to avoid stepping out of my oversized/overstuffed shoes, and pivoted on my left heel to avoid putting pressure on a very sore big toe. I wore moleskin on my glasses to reduce pressure from the nosepiece, and multiple disposable heat pads under multiple layers of clothing. I was late to work every day because I missed my turn or because I sat in my car outside the building while trying to gather enough energy to go inside. I was pale and covered in acne, with chronic infections in open cracks on my hands and feet. I slept on a couch with braces on both wrists, wearing cotton gloves over Vaseline-covered hands. I crawled on the floor when I woke up in the morning and slept for hours in a conference room at work each day. My legs gave out without warning, causing me to fall in front of strangers in public or peers at work. I carried pills to address pain, focus, and energy in one pocket, Sticky notes and a pencil to capture my thoughts in another. I was drinking alcohol at night to help me sleep and was frequently unable to eat because of sores in my mouth. I was ignoring my children, my house, and my work. The kids and I stopped visiting family and friends. We gave away our pets, and grass grew over our garden.

When I woke up, the sun was no longer overhead. I climbed into the driver's seat and drove home. Chris came home from school a few minutes later and found me standing in the kitchen with a cup of coffee.

"Hey Mom, remember this?" He waved a sheet of paper in front of me. "I don't think Kenny's car went very far, but Gret's was really fast! Mine is going to be better than both of theirs."

He had instructions for a balloon car project, the same assignment Gret and Kenny received a few years earlier. The car needed to be made from materials found around the house, and propelled only by the air in an attached balloon.

I took the sheet from Chris, thinking of the multiple runs I had made to the store for materials found "around the house" for Gret's and Kenny's projects, the trial and error of gluing soda cap wheels to juice box straw axles, then a full weekend in and out of the garage for practice runs and revisions. The masking tape to measure the travel distance was still on our garage floor.

At that moment I felt too weak to even take the two steps down into the garage.

"Let's look at it this weekend," I said.

I put the sheet on the kitchen counter with about fifty other pieces of mail and papers from school, then turned to go upstairs without looking back at Chris. I just wanted to climb into a hot bath and close my eyes.

On Saturday morning, Chris dug through the growing pile of papers and found the project sheet as I stood at the kitchen island trying to muster enough energy to make a pot of coffee.

"Hey Mom, can we work on this today? It's due on Monday."

I was shivering with cold beneath my sweatpants and winter coat, nauseous from overmedication, and struggling to focus through a fog of exhaustion and pain. I wondered if I could survive the next five minutes.

"Call your father," I said with a growl. I was furious that he had the nerve to ask anything from me.

"He's out of town," he said softly.

Chris studied the paper in his hands as he waited for my response. He looked up at me with disbelief, then genuine pain as I simply walked away.

As I drifted into and out of sleep in the tub I thought I would likely die if I didn't do something. I forced myself to go downstairs to call my doctor. As I passed the open door to the garage on my way to the kitchen I saw Kenny and Chris working on the balloon car. At least that was one thing I didn't have to worry about.

I called my primary care office and scheduled an appointment with a new doctor who had an opening right away. The waiting room was practically empty on a Saturday afternoon, and I went straight back. I was surprised because I'd shown up once before during Saturday morning walk-in hours and waited half the day to see a doctor. The weather was beautiful so I assumed people had something they'd rather do than spend a weekend afternoon at the doctor's office.

A nurse led me past my regular exam room and into one that was a mirror image on the opposite side of the hallway. I slipped into the chair and was zipping my heavy coat up to my chin when the doctor opened the door, laptop in hand. He considered me for a second, then entered the room and sat down next to me. He was young and serious, determined to review my history on the computer before talking. I watched him click and scroll, wondering what he was learning.

He turned to me and said, "So what's going on?"

I surprised myself by immediately starting to cry. "I'm miserable and exhausted. Something has to change." I didn't have the energy for details. I assumed they were in my record since I had been there so many times. Maybe this new doctor would be able to find some meaning to my chronic problems.

The doctor felt the glands in my neck and listened to my heart and lungs.

"You don't look sick," he said.

I looked down at myself and wondered what he saw. I didn't even recognize the crippled person before him. I wanted to tell him that I was energetic and fun, spontaneous and driven. All I could say was, "Something is wrong. Please help me."

He frowned at me and said, "Look, half the people who walk through that door are tired and in pain. I will give you a low dose of thyroid medication to see if that helps, but I don't think you need it."

He scribbled something on a prescription pad, tore off the top sheet and handed it to me, then walked out. His nurse came into the room seconds later to draw blood, explaining that he wanted a thyroid level check.

I filled the prescription on the way home, hopeful that it would make some difference in my energy level. The doctor called the next day, telling me that the blood test results were normal and that the medication was not needed.

The thyroid medication did seem to give me a slight increase in energy, so I took it anyway. I wondered if my thyroid was actually part of my problem, or if this was another treatment that would quickly become ineffective. If it continued to help, what would happen when I needed a refill? Would the doctor prescribe something that was clinically unnecessary? I decided to worry about that later.

I lacked the energy to continue chasing a comprehensive medical diagnosis and decided to just address each symptom as it became unbearable. I would take antibiotics for my frequent infections, surgically address joint issues, continue to drink alcohol as needed to sleep at night, and take drugs to get through the day.

I felt like I was keeping a terrible secret. I knew something was very wrong and that I was simply passing time until something disastrous happened. I thought I would suddenly drop dead and everyone would be shocked while I had been screaming "Help me!" all along. I could imagine no other outcome.

Then everything changed.

Chapter Twelve

DISCOVERY

One morning at work I was hobbling down a long corridor and eating some cookies I bought from a vending machine to try to boost my energy when I ran into my friend Prancer, so nicknamed because of a very impressive imitation of a prancing horse she'd done in her office one day.

I offered her a cookie. She took the package and read the label. "No thanks," she said. "I don't eat gluten."

She must have noticed the blank look on my face, because she explained that she was a celiac and felt much better if she avoided grains. She handed the cookies back and I quickly glanced at the label. It provided no clue to what she was talking about.

I felt uncomfortable asking for more information, so I went back to my desk and looked up "celiac" online. I learned that celiac disease was a very serious medical condition that could only be treated by following a very strict diet. Poor Prancer! She didn't seem sick to me, and I had never noticed her eating anything unusual.

The next day Prancer and I, along with many of our coworkers, attended the first of a two-day off-site meeting I had been dreading for months. I had no idea how I could stay engaged for two hours, much less two days.

I was proud that I arrived on time at the huge convention center, and found my way through the building to our ballroom. I hesitated in the doorway for a few seconds before weaving among the dozens of large, round tables toward a spot in the back corner of the room.

The room was full of energy as people talked, laughed, and jiggled ice cubes in water glasses before taking their seats. The sunlight from a wall of windows on one side of the room poured onto the thick white tablecloths and highlighted the beautiful orange and purple floral centerpieces on each table. I picked up an agenda and a folder from an empty table at the back of the room and flipped through the material. On the first day corporate leaders would provide an update on company performance and goals, then local leaders would review their business strategies on day two. I hoped I could at least get through most of the first day while leaning quietly in my dark corner.

I chewed on ice cubes to stay awake and very slowly bent and flexed my legs to avoid cramping as much as possible. I tried to pay attention to the presentations, and people-watched to distract me when I could no longer focus. I was elated that I made it to the lunch break and followed Prancer in line for the buffet. I felt sympathetic about her food limitations and was interested in what she would eat. I asked her to explain her selections as we worked our way through the options.

She didn't seem to mind educating me and described in some detail why she took the salad but not the dressing, and how she thought it was okay to eat the mayo with her sliced turkey. Yes fruit, no bread, no cookie.

Out of support for Prancer, and because I was too tired to put much thought into filling my own plate, I chose the same foods she was having. As we ate, she told me about how she had been very sick and was hospitalized when her doctor discovered she was a celiac. She was told to never eat gluten again.

Prancer explained that gluten was a protein found in several grains and added to many common foods. Eating at home was easy for her because she knew what brands were gluten-free and could check labels when she was shopping. Eating out, where food was prepared out of sight and labels were not available, was much more difficult. Fresh meats, fruits, and vegetables were generally safe since they didn't naturally contain gluten, but she had to be careful that gluten might have been added in sauces or seasonings.

The way fresh foods were handled could also present a risk. Even gluten-free foods made her sick if they contacted a surface, utensil, or container that was not well cleaned after contact with a food containing gluten. Because of the risk of this cross-contamination, she was cautious about eating in restaurants, buying foods packaged in a common area such as a grocery store deli, or eating food from buffet lines.

I stared at the lump of mayonnaise scooped from a family-style bowl and the couple of grapes remaining on her plate. She told me that over the years through trial and error she learned the types of food preparation or sharing situations that were generally okay and the ones to avoid. She thought that today everything would be fine.

Our lunch break ended and I returned to the back of the room, thinking about what would happen if there was gluten in something Prancer ate. I remembered a news article about a child with a peanut allergy who went into anaphylactic shock after giving a high five to another child who had eaten a peanut butter bar. I wondered if a celiac's sensitivity to gluten was similar to a peanut allergy. Would they have an anaphylactic reaction if they were exposed? Were celiacs allergic to gluten? The kids' schools regularly shared information about nut allergies and efforts to protect affected students, but nothing about protecting individuals sensitive to gluten. Gluten issues must not be very common, or maybe only adults develop this condition?

The next thing I knew the speakers were wrapping up for the day. I'd made it! I felt like I'd just won a gold medal in a fierce competition and wanted to jump onto a table and shout "YES!!" to celebrate my victory. I actually was exhausted and shaky, but highly encouraged and greatly satisfied by my success in completing a full day of doing what was expected of me just like everyone else.

Intrigued by Prancer's story and naturally curious about her diet, I decided to eat gluten-free foods for the next couple of meals at home. Thinking that fresh chicken was okay since we ate turkey for lunch, I baked a couple of chicken breasts for my dinner. I didn't think I should use any breading and had no idea what sauces or seasonings were allowed, so I ate the chicken completely plain. I considered having some of the mashed potatoes and applesauce the kids were eating but didn't know if they would be on Prancer's diet. I didn't see gluten listed on the package labels, but I didn't see gluten listed on the bread package either, and I knew bread was not on the diet. The next morning I drank a cup of coffee with bacon and eggs, which I thought would be okay since I saw Prancer eating them before at a breakfast meeting. I skipped the toast.

I took my regular spot at the back of the room as we began our second day of meetings, feeling a little more rested and a little less achy than the day before.

During lunch break in the buffet line, I again chose sliced turkey and fruit but passed on the salad since I found it difficult to eat without dressing. Seated on a wooden folding chair, about ten minutes into the meal I realized that I wasn't restless and anxious to stand up as I had been while eating the day before.

Wait, my back didn't hurt! I felt no spasms, no stabbing pain. I leaned to the left, then the right. I tapped my feet on the floor. No reaction!

What was going on? Was this because of Prancer's diet? No, that wasn't possible. Was it? Could eating more of something - poultry, maybe -improve the effect of my pain medicine?

For the rest of the afternoon I remained on the chair, cautiously shifting my weight to test my back muscles. No cramping!

When I caught up with Prancer at the end of the day, everyone was dashing out. It was Friday evening and well into rush hour. Traffic would be terrible. Prancer patiently listened to my raving, then calmly suggested that I remain on the diet through the weekend to continue the experiment.

I did continue through the weekend and the following week. I shed several layers of much-too-warm clothing, my skin began to clear up, and my joint pain, cramps, and body aches went away. By the end of the week I was beginning to realize that the turn in my health was real.

I woke up on Saturday morning to bright daylight and was immediately disoriented, since I hadn't been able to sleep through the night in years. I was totally relaxed, and the pillows that should have been carefully tucked all around me to prevent movement as I slept were strewn all over the floor. My back was perfectly calm and pain-free, and I could move my legs. And I was flat on my back!

I looked up at the ceiling and smiled, and then laughed so hard that after a while I rolled onto my side and pulled my knees up to my chest.

Then I began to cry. Hard, heavy sobs. Relief and joy and surprise and disbelief that all my years of struggling with my health might have been avoided.

Because of my diet?! Was everything because of my diet?? IT'S JUST FOOD!!

I gasped for breath as my mind caught up with my emotions. Did food cause me to have arthritis, or was arthritis a misdiagnosis? Did I have celiac disease? Was having cancer somehow related to all of this? Can being a celiac give you cancer? Did food give me cancer?

I had so many questions. I needed to understand what was going on, and I needed to find more to eat than plain meat and fruit. If gluten was my problem, it would never cross my lips again no matter what I had to do to avoid it. I would happily eat rocks for every meal if that's what it took to be healthy and reclaim my life!

I was still having difficulty believing that anything had changed. I rose from the couch and walked across the room. I stood barefoot in the shower and let the water run down my face, trying to wrap my mind around what was happening. Every thought and every ounce of energy just a few days before were focused on my very sick body. And now my problems had suddenly evaporated?

Of course I was overjoyed, but also very deeply disturbed in a way I had never been by any of my health concerns. How could something so fundamental as eating, which I'd thought absolutely nothing about, have such a profound impact my life? If this was real, then how, in thirty years of declining health, did I never once have any indication that food was the cause?

Because it's *FOOD!* The food pyramid does not have an asterisk with a footnote explaining that one of the basic food groups might be harmful to some people without their knowledge. Nobody turns down cake at a birthday party or bread at a restaurant because it causes joint pain and confusion. No one worries about developing muscle cramps or crippling exhaustion when they take candy from a jar or plunge their hand into a bowl of chips at a party. No alternatives are offered to donuts and bagels at a school celebration or early sports practice, no substitutes for pasta and sandwiches are available at lunch meetings. Nobody ever considers that someone cannot eat these things. Ever! If food could cause such significant issues, wouldn't people be talking about it? Wouldn't doctors be looking for it?

I'd been eating bread and cookies and pasta my entire life. Wouldn't I have known if they were making me sick? And if food was making me sick, shouldn't that diagnosis come from a physician or be the result of some advanced clinical testing? Did I make a life-changing discovery by accident, just by deciding one day to eat what my friend was eating? Was my life completely subject to chance?

Eventually I settled down and began my quest to learn more about celiac disease and gluten. The history was very long! A Greek doctor first identified the relationship between food and the symptoms of celiac disease thousands of years ago, but he could never figure out which foods were causing the problems. Physicians in the late 1800s discovered that celiacs improved when starches were eliminated from their diet, but the true cause of celiac disease symptoms was not determined until World War Two. The health of Dutch children with celiac disease improved when bread was not available during the war, then deteriorated when bread was returned to their diets. Doctors made the connection to gluten, which prompted further research, leading to a greater understanding of the disease.

We now know that when celiacs eat gluten their immune systems react by destroying villi, tiny hairlike structures in the small intestine. Celiac disease is described as an autoimmune disorder because of the abnormal immune response to gluten, and a digestive disease because the damage to the intestinal villi prevents proper absorption of nutrients from food. The classic symptom is diarrhea, but abdominal pain and bloating are also very frequent complaints.

As I read, I flashed back to torturous forty-five-minute bus rides during grade school with sweat pouring down my face as I tried desperately to avoid soiling my pants, and my brother and me performing our regular after-dinner routine of pressing our chests into the carpet while sticking our butts in the air in an attempt to pass gas and alleviate the horrible pain and pressure in our upper abdomens. This butt elevation method was common practice for us, which we initiated only if half an hour of forced burping didn't reduce our hugely swollen bellies. And we were a couple of skinny kids. We were branded as having "sensitive" stomachs, and fed paregoric to reduce our pain and discomfort. I don't remember anything about the effectiveness of this narcotic, only the terrible smell and taste of the clear liquid from a brown glass bottle. I hadn't thought about that in years.

As an adult, I occasionally had an intestinal reaction to food, but nothing that raised any red flags. I knew I couldn't eat heavy, creamy dishes such as spinach and artichoke dip at Joe's Crab Shack (details omitted in an attempt to preserve dignity), and that I was much more comfortable if I didn't eat anything before boarding the metro train to work. Breakfast didn't always upset my stomach, but inconsistency and an inability to identify a specific cause worried me enough to skip a morning meal when restroom availability was limited.

The number of medications available to treat upset stomach and diarrhea convinced me that digestive issues were common and that my challenges were not unusual. I never considered that manageable digestive problems were cause for concern. I thought you simply avoided what bothered you or treated your symptoms.

Looking back with my new knowledge of celiac disease allowed me to see a chronic pattern in my history I hadn't recognized before. The pattern became even more clear as I read an article distinguishing celiac disease symptoms in children and adults. Digestive symptoms are seen in most celiac children, but less than half of adults. Adults may exhibit any number of a long list of symptoms, including many I had experienced: fatigue, joint pain, skin rash, arthritis, tingling and pain in the hands and feet, mouth sores, weakness, and trouble concentrating. It seemed very strange that so many seemingly unrelated issues could be caused by the same disease!

Celiac disease was identified as "common," affecting more than three million people in the United States. Most people with celiac disease either don't know they have it or have been misdiagnosed with another condition, with ten years or more often needed to diagnose an adult celiac. For every celiac diagnosed, 140 are misdiagnosed, and 45 percent of celiacs are identified as hypochondriacs prior to their diagnosis.

I wanted to slam my fists down in frustration when I read about this delay in diagnosis, because of the needless suffering it caused for so many people. But I acknowledged that doctors would have difficulty recognizing the relationship between a wide range of symptoms if they weren't very familiar with the disease. Each symptom individually could easily indicate something else.

Who were the celiac medical experts who finally made accurate diagnoses, and how did a patient find these people? I wondered if I would eventually run into one on the course I was taking.

I discovered research showing that the longer a person with celiac disease goes undiagnosed, the greater the chance of having another autoimmune disease such as rheumatoid arthritis. Does that mean that celiacs develop another autoimmune disease because they have a flawed immune system, or does their flawed immune system express different symptoms at different times, resulting in multiple diagnoses based on the system or body part affected at the time?

While I still had many unanswered questions, I was more confident in my realization that celiac disease was a known condition that could explain my chronic health issues as well as my improved health since eliminating gluten.

The next step was to remove gluten from my diet permanently.

Chapter Thirteen

READING LABELS

O ff I went to the store, eager to expand my options and find which of the foods from my regular grocery list I would be able to eat. My goal was to avoid wheat, rye, and barley, the grains containing gluten.

I headed straight for the produce. I knew I could eat all the fresh fruits and vegetables I wanted. At the end of the first aisle was a display of ketchup, our regular brand and an item on my list. I picked up a bottle and flipped it around to check the ingredients. Tomato concentrate, vinegar, corn syrup, salt, spice, onion powder, natural flavoring. That looks okay, doesn't it? No gluten-containing grains listed.

Wait, what is natural flavoring? Didn't Prancer tell me gluten is sometimes a hidden ingredient in flavorings? Hmm. . . I picked up another brand of ketchup, and then another, finding similar ingredients. I searched entire labels for all the brands, front and back, looking for definitive information about gluten but didn't see anything. I put a bottle in the cart, and a question mark next to "ketchup" on my list. The kids could eat it, but I wasn't sure if I should.

On the next aisle I noticed that taco seasoning and taco shells were clearly marked gluten-free. Woohoo! Not on my list, but into the cart they went. They would be nice additions to my current diet. Interesting that I never noticed "gluten-free" in big letters on the box of taco shells I regularly kept in my pantry.

A can of sloppy joe sauce caught my eye and I thought about how good sloppy joes would taste even without the forbidden bun. The sauce label was not conclusive. It lacked a gluten-free statement and listed ingredients basically the same as ketchup. "Natural flavor" again.

I realized that the device in my hand gave me the ability to resolve my uncertainty, and I searched "Is sloppy joe sauce gluten-free?" on my cell phone. The manufacturer's website clearly stated that the sauce was gluten-free. But it contained distilled vinegar, and someone posted that they called the manufacturer and their distilled vinegar is derived from either wheat or corn. Diving farther into links about vinegar, I read that distilled vinegar could be made from wheat, but the gluten is removed during the distillation process.

Okay, that was a little complicated but the manufacturer's statement was pretty clear: gluten-free. It seemed weird to consider eating something I knew was made from wheat, but if the gluten was truly gone there was no problem, right? I put the sloppy joe sauce in the cart and I looked at it for a second, trying hard to override my emotional resistance with a scientific argument that the sauce would be okay for me to eat.

I almost cheered as I moved to the next aisle and saw "gluten-free" boldly stated on the jar of my favorite brand of peanut butter. Peanut butter and jelly made a perfect sandwich in my opinion, and was a staple I hoped to bring back to my lunch once I found the gluten-free bread Prancer recommended.

Jelly was unfortunately not so clearly marked, so I picked up jars one by one and inspected our favorite varieties. At the end of the ingredients list orange marmalade said "contains wheat." I unconsciously wiped my hand on my shirt after putting it back on the shelf. Grape went into the cart after I found the words "gluten-free" on the back label. Strawberry preserves, my favorite, were described online by the manufacturer as having "no gluten-containing ingredients."

No gluten-containing ingredients. Does that mean gluten-free? One celiac support group warned of the risk of contamination with this product, since it was manufactured on equipment that processes other products that do contain gluten. Prancer mentioned cross-contamination as a serious concern. Wasn't this something I should worry about too?

I put the preserves back on the shelf and checked the other two brands, finding similar results. Feeling a twinge of disappointment, I tried to envision my ridiculously early Tuesday mornings without my favorite quick breakfast.

Kenny practiced with the jazz band several days a week before school. On the days I drove for the car pool I relished ten minutes of calm and quiet with a cup of coffee and a toasted bagel covered in melting cream cheese with huge chunks of cold strawberry preserves piled precariously high on top before I filled my car with rambunctious teenage boys. If I could find gluten-free bagels I would try them with boring grape jelly, but it wouldn't be the same.

I attempted to shake off my emotional attachment to the strawberry preserves, and moved to the canned goods section where I expected most of the items to be gluten-free. Corn, green beans, and peaches were identified online as "naturally gluten-free" by their manufacturers, and one stated that their products would only be labeled gluten-free if they were tested for the presence of gluten.

Ah, so maybe that was the story for ketchup too. Maybe it didn't contain gluten, but had not been tested and so was not labeled gluten-free. Or maybe it actually contained gluten.

How could I tell the difference between gluten-free products that were not labeled, products that actually contained gluten as a "hidden ingredient," and products that would be gluten-free but contained gluten due to cross-contamination? I didn't see any warnings about my specific canned goods online, so I put them in my cart and started to move on, then hesitated and added a question mark next to each item on my list.

Every one of my favorite soups and our regular brand of pork and beans contained wheat. Tuna was "naturally gluten-free" with no warnings about cross-contamination. Apparently the tuna was not tested, since it wasn't labeled gluten-free, but maybe that was okay. I tried to imagine a fish canning process and measure the possibility of gluten exposure, but I truly had no idea. I discovered that some canned fish did list wheat on the label, so clearly gluten was sometimes present in fish production. I made a small groaning sound as I put tuna in the cart and entered a question mark on my list.

I wasn't doing a great job of evaluating food for my new diet, and I thought I should assess my strategy. Should I assume that a product is safe if it did not actually contain gluten, or assume nothing was safe unless it was labeled gluten-free?

Buying only items labeled gluten-free felt like the safer thing to do, but then would I be unnecessarily excluding products that were gluten-free but not tested? I thought maybe I should simply eat plain meat and fresh fruit for the rest of my life. That would have been much better than making myself sick or worrying about every bite I put in my mouth!

In the interest of avoiding a panic attack in the same grocery store where I'd once collapsed into a sweaty heap on the floor, I decided to finish shopping the way I started. I would check labels and exclude items that clearly contained gluten, and make a note for the ones I wasn't sure about. I could do more research at home.

I took a deep breath and picked up a package of mashed potatoes. I was shocked to see more than twenty ingredients listed on the package, but fortunately none was wheat, barley, or rye. I searched the manufacturer's website but couldn't find specific information about gluten. I stood looking at the package, unsure whether I should put it in the cart or back on the shelf. Unsure equals no, or unsure equals yes? Arghhh! In the cart. The kids could eat it.

Moving through the store and down my list I discovered that our regular brands of granola bars, rice cereal, rice cereal treats, and flavored chips all definitely contained gluten, while yogurt, fruit snacks, soda, and plain chips definitely did not. Oatmeal, our favorite smoked almonds, cheese, and ground beef were questionable due to cross-contamination.

I found that coffee did not naturally contain gluten and was unlikely to be contaminated, but some celiacs experienced a reaction to coffee due to cross-reactivity. The proteins in coffee are very similar to those in gluten, so the immune system gets confused and reacts to coffee as it does when gluten is consumed. Uh, okay.

I examined the bag of coffee in my hand. Did I have to give up coffee? I was drinking coffee during the experiment with Prancer's diet, and that went well! I would keep cross-reactivity in mind, but put the bag of coffee in my cart anyway. I would have to think about that one.

Prancer told me that all animal protein is naturally gluten-free unless gluten is added when seasoned, breaded, or marinated. Eggs are an animal protein, right? I checked to be sure they were in the same category, and learned that very sensitive celiacs report problems eating eggs from chickens fed a diet heavy with grains. Wow.

I seemed to be okay, and I had been eating eggs. Maybe I wasn't supersensitive? I wondered how I could tell what the chickens were fed when they produced the eggs. I didn't see anything on the carton. Feeding chickens something other than grains seemed odd. What else would they eat? I'd heard of grass-fed beef, but never grass-fed chickens.

As I pondered whether it would be cruel to make a chicken eat grass, I put the eggs in my cart and put chicken diets on a list of questions to resolve when I had more time. I was too tired to think about it. I had been in the store for three and a half hours and considered more than one hundred items. Thirty-eight clearly contained gluten, twenty-one were identified as gluten-free, and fifty-five were inconclusive.

I looked into my cart, disheartened by the small number of items I was sure I could eat and concerned that several of the foods I had been eating to avoid gluten were questionable. Did that make sense? Could I feel better but still be making my body sick?

As I struggled to educate myself about food labeling, manufacturing practices, and safe levels of gluten exposure, we discovered that the kids also benefited from a gluten-free diet. It started with them as a curiosity, as it had with me, but they committed to avoiding gluten when they experienced drastic improvements in how they felt.

Kenny had suffered from back pain so severe at sixteen he couldn't sit on the bleachers at school, and Chris received treatment for anxiety that started when he was two. Gretchen and Chris both endured frequent intense headaches, and multiple physicians had been unable to discover the cause.

When they eliminated gluten, Kenny's back pain went away and Chris's anxiety improved so significantly he no longer required any of his three prescribed medications. Gret and Chris's headaches disappeared, and all three felt unexpected relief from fatigue, brain fog, stomach sensitivities, and body aches. Kenny gained weight, Gret and Chris lost weight, and they all stopped waking up multiple times during the night.

We learned that someone is ten times more likely to have celiac disease if an immediate family member has it. Maybe celiac disease explained the kids' improved symptoms on a gluten- free diet and could account for Gret's diagnosis at age seventeen of Hashimoto's disease, a thyroid disorder strongly connected with celiac disease and most often diagnosed in women more than twice her age.

It sounds ridiculous in retrospect, but even after my own epiphany I don't think I would have related any of the kids' issues to food if I hadn't seen firsthand the effects of changing their diet.

I felt intense pressure to immediately provide plenty of satisfying food and to be able to definitively answer every question the kids had about what they should eat. This fierce need to protect my children was unlike anything I had encountered since they were infants. I guess they seemed vulnerable to me, and I thought I was the only one who could help them. I certainly didn't want to send them down the path of health challenges I had been on for most of my life if it could be avoided.

Almost everything the kids had been eating their entire lives needed to be replaced. I took a few days off work for more research and exploration, and found hundreds of products that were gluten-free through published lists from manufacturers, grocery stores, and celiac support groups. I discovered a section of a local grocery store dedicated to gluten-free foods, and an app I could use to identify gluten-free items. We were able to replace most of our regular diet with gluten-free substitutes and felt much more confident in our choices. I also learned that the FDA would soon finalize a rule to regulate the use of "gluten-free" labeling that would make shopping much easier.

In the middle of our diet transition, a dozen members of Gretchen's ultimate Frisbee college team spent the night at our house. A big two-day tournament was held nearby, and there was not enough time for the team to drive back to school between late night and early morning games. Sleeping bags, inflatable mattresses, backpacks, and gym bags covered our basement floor.

I removed every item containing gluten from our pantry, cabinets, and shelves and placed them on our kitchen table and island. The girls happily loaded everything into grocery bags to take back to school, and we were well on our way to a gluten-free house.

As I peered into our relatively bare pantry and contemplated the widespread presence of gluten in our fairly typical American diet, I finally realized why I felt no pain in my entire body after my first neck surgery. The puzzle must have been sitting in the back of my mind unsolved for years. It finally made sense.

When my allergic reaction to the new pain medication caused my throat to swell and prevented me from eating, I wasn't exposed to any gluten for a couple of days and my pain went away. It was the same drastic change that occurred when I eliminated gluten on Prancer's diet; I just didn't recognize what was happening at the time. I took a minute to appreciate that second chance and wondered how many other people discovered a sensitivity to gluten through a similar unintentional method.

The kids and I anticipated limited options and difficulty finding foods we wanted to eat on our new gluten-free diet, but we didn't realize the integral role food played in our lives until we had to consider everything we put in our mouths and plan what we were going to eat everywhere we went. Eating was no longer a spontaneous act. We couldn't grab lunch from the cafeteria, get snacks at a gas station, or pick up fast food during a busy day of running errands. We either took food with us when we went out, or researched restaurants in advance for gluten- free options and their ability to avoid cross-contamination.

We did get "glutened" a few times, sometimes the result of an overly optimistic attitude; others came as a total surprise. Exposure to gluten affected us all dramatically, causing body aches, vomiting, diarrhea, headaches, and an inability to focus. Eventually we identified restaurants at all price levels with knowledgeable staff and effective practices for consistently providing gluten-free dishes, so we seldom went anywhere else. The risk of losing the ability to function normally for days or even weeks greatly dampened our previously adventurous approach to new food experiences.

Our first "muffin Monday" morning without fresh blueberry

and chocolate chip muffins revealed an emotional attachment to food that surprised us all. We slowly uncovered a lifetime of food-related family traditions that would never be the same. We would no longer get piping hot funnel cakes at the fair and spend the rest of the afternoon licking sugar from our lips. We wouldn't go to the donut shop to pick out bagels and donuts for an early morning road trip or visit the ice cream shop to select a birthday cake from their glossy photos and flavor menus. There would be no s'mores at the fire pit or hot tomato soup with grilled cheese sandwiches on a cold winter day, no hot dogs at the baseball game, no cinnamon pretzels dipped in frosting while Christmas shopping at the mall. We would no longer seize every Pillsbury sugar cookie design as it arrived in stores, eating more raw cookies than baked, and arguing about which color dough tasted the best (orange pumpkins, no doubt). We were reminded again and again that these small things that played a big role in our lives were forever changed.

The kids and I were a tight little team, sharing information about our experiences and supporting each other in our efforts to learn and to find new and better things to eat. We constantly discussed restaurant experiences, good and bad, as well as recipes and new brands of gluten-free bread, pasta, snacks, and frozen meals. Outside our little group, though, things were different. People didn't understand what we were doing or why.

One of many difficult scenarios played out during a big family gathering for Thanksgiving, when Grandma plopped a huge serving of her signature stuffing on my plate with obvious pride.

"I know you love this stuffing!" she said, with a wink and a kiss on my cheek.

I stared at my plate for a second, then looked up at Grandma, aching with sympathy.

"Remember, Grandma, I told you that bread makes me sick?" I asked in little more than a whisper. "This stuffing has toast, right?"

Grandma looked at the dish in her hand. "But I made it just the way you like it, with lots of bacon. Surely you can have just a few bites!"

I felt everyone's eyes on me.

"I'm sorry, Grandma," I said softly. "It looks great. But I'm afraid it will make me really sick if I eat it."

Grandma turned away with her head down like I had broken her heart. Everyone at the table looked at me like I was pure evil for upsetting Grandma on Thanksgiving after all of her hard work. My stomach knotted with shame. I wanted to disappear. I filled a new plate with ham and turkey and wished for anyone to start talking about anything other than food.

We experienced this type of Grandma situation again and again. The disappointment was palpable when I didn't sample a coworker's winning entry at the annual chili cook-off or when the kids didn't eat a slice of pizza at a friend's party. We felt that we were truly insulting people when we didn't share what they were eating or accept food they made for us. We understood, and imagined feeling the same way!

Chris took a gourmet cooking class at school and brought home creations he knew from the start none of us could eat. He was still clearly disappointed when actually faced with the fact that we wouldn't sample and comment on something he'd made from scratch.

We regularly discussed how to handle these ongoing challenges and found that we all sometimes took risks with food to avoid an awkward social situation. I don't think any of us ever ate something we knew would make us sick, but at first we all ate things we didn't want to eat. I remember scraping a gravy made of who knows what off a steak at a formal award banquet and trying to take a few bites from the middle rather than ordering a special plate or trying to explain to a table of strangers why I wasn't eating. The kids went out with friends and made their best guess about what might be safe from a restaurant menu they didn't have an opportunity to review in advance.

Over time we learned what to expect from other people and how to handle a variety of situations, but I don't think the social aspects of eating differently became any easier. We didn't want to stand out, and we didn't want to disappoint other people or make anyone feel uncomfortable. But we felt great on our new diet, so we were willing to face the challenges necessary to avoid gluten. We did our best to explain what we were doing and why to people around us. We also sometimes moved food around on a plate to look like we were eating it, and exchanged a full plate with a friend for an empty one so we weren't obviously avoiding food at a party.

Maybe that was just me.

Chapter Fourteen

PROFESSIONAL HELP

The change in my health was remarkable but not complete. I was still taking lots of prescription medications for pain and focus, and thought something must be wrong if I continued to need that support. If I tried taking a smaller dose or waited longer between doses I was miserable. Plus, sometimes I felt terrible for no apparent reason. I experienced back and joint pain as well as paralyzing weakness exactly like the symptoms I felt before eliminating gluten from my diet.

My research showed that the most common reason for ongoing celiac symptoms on a gluten-free diet was incomplete adherence to a gluten-free diet. This seemed entirely plausible in my case, since I could identify a long list of ways I might be exposed to gluten. A number of the questions I had while grocery shopping, such as labeling and cross-contamination, were not completely resolved and remained areas of possible risk.

My primary concern had to do with the amount of gluten in gluten-free products. There were no standard testing requirements for a product to be labeled gluten-free; instead, the assessment practice was at the discretion of the manufacturer. If the manufacturer's method was flawed or unreliable, products containing gluten could still bear a gluten-free label. Also, analytical equipment was not able to detect very low levels of gluten, so *all* products labeled gluten-free could contain some gluten. If I was one of the "highly sensitive" celiacs, even gluten levels of twenty parts per million (the allowable limit for gluten-free products under the draft FDA rule) could cause problems.

Cross-contamination was also high on my list of concerns, particularly processing of gluten-free products in an area where gluten is also handled. To avoid contamination, each staff member would have to receive training and consistently follow safe practices, such as thoroughly cleaning all equipment and surfaces and changing gloves after handling products with gluten. Most people I knew had never heard of gluten, so I wasn't superconfident about the level of awareness in food processing. Residual gluten in my kitchen was another source of potential exposure. I replaced our toaster, griddle, wooden utensils, and cutting board, but not everything in the kitchen. Maybe I missed something important.

The apps I relied on to identify gluten-free products were an additional risk. Manufacturing practices and suppliers often change, so a product that is gluten-free at one time may not be the next. I had no idea who updated the apps and how often, so the information I relied on to guide my purchases could have been outdated and inaccurate.

My concerns made sense, I thought, except that the kids were fine. If I was exposed to gluten because of one of these risks, wouldn't they be affected too? They had no health complaints, and when they did have symptoms they could always identify the cause. I wasn't eating any differently than they were. Was I just more sensitive? I thought maybe if I was super- sensitive I might be reacting to chicken or eggs because of the grains fed to the chickens. Or maybe I was reacting to coffee because of that similarity in protein structure between coffee and gluten. The kids didn't drink coffee, so they wouldn't be affected by cross-reactivity.

The list of possibilities was long, and I didn't know how to figure out what was causing my problems. Maybe I was bothered by something I hadn't even thought about. I believed my health was dependent on eating the right foods (or avoiding the wrong ones), so my inability to understand and manage the factors controlling my health was both frustrating and frightening. The endless research required to decide what to eat and what to avoid was completely overwhelming, and rarely conclusive. I needed help.

I searched for professionals to resolve my uncertainties and was excited to find a doctor nearby who specialized in food sensitivities and immunological diseases. What a perfect combination! His experience was impressive, and he was rated a top doctor in his field. I was confident he would know how to address my questions and provide direction.

In the only occupied office of a new professional building, the doctor called me from the waiting room himself and greeted me with a warm handshake like he was genuinely happy to see me. He was a jolly-looking man with a round face and pink cheeks. In the exam room, he sat facing me with no distracting computer or papers and listened carefully as I chronicled my health history since high school. I described my procedures over the years and the effects of pain and exhaustion on my life.

I recounted my discovery of gluten with great enthusiasm and explained how its absence changed me. Just as my mind switched gears from storytelling to asking for the help I needed to move forward, the doctor's entire demeanor changed. He jumped up and threw his hands into the air.

"Everything is 'gluten' these days," he yelled, pacing the room. "It's ridiculous! You have been brainwashed by commercialism!"

I sat, stunned, not sure what to do next.

"Why would I feel so much better after eliminating gluten?" I asked, genuinely curious.

"Your health history includes rheumatoid arthritis, and you should expect flare-ups and unpredictability," he said. "Pain medication and anti-inflammatories are more effective on some days than others."

"I don't understand," I said. "I have more energy, I'm sleeping better, and I don't have body aches since changing my diet."

His entire face flushed dark red and he screeched, "Gluten. Is. Not. POISON!!!" He panted a little, then returned to his seat. With exaggerated patience he asked, "You had a colonoscopy, right? Did the doctor who performed your procedure say you were a celiac? If you were a celiac it would have shown up during the colonoscopy. Do you know how many factors can affect your sleep? Alcohol consumption, pets in your bed, exercise, light levels, the use of electronics at bedtime."

I was intimidated by his passion and disheartened by my failure to convince him to take my story seriously. After a few more exchanges, I had pretty much given up on his ability to help me, but realized I didn't know who could.

"I'm sorry to upset you," I said. "But I know I am eating something that is making me sick and I don't know how to figure out what it is. What kind of doctor should I go to next for help?"

At this point he was at the door and reaching for the handle. He turned around and glared at me for what seemed like forever. I actually felt a flash of adrenaline as I realized I had no way out. I wasn't really afraid of him, but his unpredictable behavior put me on edge.

"I guess I could run some tests," he said, then walked out the door.

His nurse came into the room almost immediately to draw blood for food allergy testing.

I still felt dazed and distracted half an hour later as I stood in the checkout line at the grocery store. I was jolted by a call from the doctor, who asked permission to run some antibody tests on the blood they collected.

A few days later he called to tell me that the only positive food allergy reaction was to eggs, but lots of people have that reaction and eat eggs every day without problems. He said he ran a test for celiac disease and it was negative.

"Don't worry about it," he said. "You are fine. Eat normally."

Well, that was confusing and not at all helpful.

Was there any action for me to take? Did I learn that I was allergic to eggs but should go ahead and eat them because other people do without problems? What about the negative celiac test? Should I be concerned about the implications of that result?

My experience with the doctor was so bizarre, I didn't feel like I connected with him so didn't have a strong reaction to his findings. But he was an expert in food and immunology. And he conducted analytical testing.

I learned through internet research that there were many inconclusive celiac tests. But he didn't say inconclusive. He said "negative." Since I had no idea which test he performed I didn't really know the value of the results.

I certainly wasn't going to "eat normally." Did he really think that was useful guidance? I was trying to figure out what was causing symptoms, not convince myself that my old diet was fine. I wished we could have had a more meaningful discussion about the effects of food on the body and what could be causing my symptoms. I really wanted to understand what was going on.

I was right back where I started and felt a little less enthusiastic about telling my story to another health professional. Still, I decided to ask my primary care doctor for advice. I now had my gluten discovery experience to share and specific questions to ask. With the new knowledge that my health issues were food-based, maybe he would know what kind of specialist could help me. I also wanted to ask him why celiac disease wasn't detected during my colonoscopy. Was it even possible to detect celiac disease during a colonoscopy? I thought the villi destroyed by celiac disease were in the small intestine, near the stomach. Would they have been seen with a scope inserted from, well, the other end of the body? How long is that scope?

I requested the results from the new food allergy testing so I could discuss them with my doctor. When I received a hard copy in the mail, I was surprised to find five pages of information. I was showing a strong allergic reaction to a number of trees, grasses, and molds. No shock there, since I knew I was allergic to pretty much everything. Just months earlier I developed welts when I brushed against a live Christmas tree.

I showed no allergic reaction to a list of about thirty foods, including grains, nuts, meats, and gluten. No shock there either. By then I knew that celiacs have an abnormal, destructive auto-immune reaction to gluten, which is different than an exaggerated but normal allergic reaction to gluten. A negative allergy test did not mean that I wasn't a celiac.

I was stunned by abnormal thyroid antibody levels that suggested that my immune system was attacking my thyroid, and elevated antinuclear antibodies further attesting to an immune system attack on my own tissues. On the last page of the report I found the statement "no serological evidence of celiac disease" with a note warning that the test was not appropriate for individuals with celiac disease who maintain a gluten-free diet. Okay, so that explained the negative celiac test, but what was going on with my immune system?

My primary care doctor didn't really show any interest in my gluten story or my self-diagnosis of celiac disease, but he was concerned about my autoimmune activity. He repeated the antibody tests, with similar results.

In a follow-up visit he told me that test results are frequently abnormal even when there is no underlying disease, but since I continued to have symptoms I should see a rheumatologist.

While the referral to a rheumatologist was absolutely appropriate, it was like a bucket of ice water thrown in my face. The fear and darkness I experienced with my breast cancer diagnosis suddenly flooded over me and I felt like I was being tossed into a dark pit of known horrors. My heart raced and I was overwhelmed by a desire to run. I thought I might throw up.

I vaguely recognized that there were no hands gripping me to drag me away and that I pretty much had complete control over what was happening. I took the list of recommended rheumatologists from the physician, said thanks, and walked out of the office.

In my car, hands shaking, I looked at the referral slip. I was surprised by such a strong reaction to my doctor's recommendation. My mind clearly associated rheumatologists with immunosuppressants and the increased risk of cancer when taking them. I reminded myself that I was in control of next steps, and that consulting with a rheumatologist wouldn't increase my risk of anything.

My latest test results identified two new autoimmune conditions. This information hijacked me emotionally and made it difficult for me to resist the pull toward the medical practice of diagnosis and treatment that I had experienced my whole life. I felt a strong need to take my results to a specialist, discuss the diagnosis, and receive a treatment plan that would bring my test results into a normal range. That might feel like success, and was the approach accepted and expected by every physician who ever treated me.

But when I thought about it rationally, I knew what I truly needed was different. I needed to figure out what was causing my body to react and to generate abnormal test results, not control or mask the reaction. I truly believed food was the key to my fate and if I could just get help figuring out what to eat, all the test results would return to normal and I would be fine.

Okay, so I convinced myself to disregard the standard course of action and take ownership for my medical journey. Great. A unique path. How does one go about defining the moves in uncharted territory?

All I could do was to take one step at a time with the goal to focus on the cause of my symptoms and not get sidetracked by emotion or habit.

I decided against scheduling the next appointment with a rheumatologist, since I didn't think it would help. The rheumatologist who treated me initially was a highly rated physician and a researcher in the fields of arthritis and immunology. From the first visit onward our discussions were limited to the prescribed treatment and testing regimen, never about possible causes of my condition other than the likelihood of a genetic risk factor that was outside my control. I thought it was unlikely that a new doctor would deviate from this convention.

Chapter Fifteen

GLIMMER OF HOPE

While working to determine my next move, I learned that internal medicine doctors specialize in disease prevention and complex illnesses. Cautiously optimistic, I scheduled an appointment with one who subspecialized in immunology. He listened to my story and told me to begin eating grains immediately. They are a staple and should never be removed from the diet no matter what.

I began to think that I misunderstood the concept of immunology and was exaggerating the ability of a specialist in that field to help me with my dilemma. I would try a different approach.

Since a gastroenterologist specializes in the digestive tract and its disorders, I thought I would give that a try next. The doctor I saw, a big guy who looked like he could have played professional football, carried out a less animated but no less passionate version of the food sensitivity doctor's rant.

"Far too many people are eliminating essential fiber from their diets for absolutely no reason," he said. "Reintroduce grains to your diet as soon as you leave this office. Celiac disease is a rare and serious condition, but the only conclusive diagnosis is based on direct observation of damaged villi in the small intestine. Circumstantial evidence is worthless and ridiculous. If you are adamant about pursuing a change to the normal diet that has sustained humans for thousands of years, eat gluten every day for three months and then schedule an endoscopy so I can check your villi. Performing an endoscopy when gluten is not present in the diet is pointless since the villi will recover and appear normal."

I sat quietly as I considered three months of gluten hell, imagining my inability to function due to pain, exhaustion, and confusion. I struggled for the words that would effectively communicate my serious concerns about further irritating my already self-destructive immune system and that would express my need for assurance that the procedure was necessary and worth the sacrifice.

The doctor seemed unaffected by my hesitation. "I am very busy but can probably find a slot on my calendar in about three months for the procedure. My scheduler will be in to talk to you about timing and preparation. Once my diagnosis is complete, my office will provide the education you need for any required diet changes."

The doctor headed out of the room. Anxious to slow a plan I did not yet support, I told his back that I was worried about eating gluten, since I knew it made me sick.

He turned from the hallway with a smirk. "Exactly. Most people aren't willing to do what it takes for a conclusive diagnosis."

I abandoned my attempts to quickly formulate logical questions about the effect and necessity of returning gluten to my diet, and asked the only clear question that came to mind.

"What is the treatment if an endoscopy proves I'm a celiac?"

"Lifelong elimination of gluten is the only treatment for celiac disease," he stated dully, then walked away.

His scheduler suddenly appeared in the exam room. Distracted and frustrated, I told her I wasn't prepared to schedule the procedure but would call her back after checking my work calendar. I don't know why I said that. I guess I just needed time to think. She left immediately, but I stayed behind to consider my options.

I was committed to a lifelong elimination of gluten from my

diet. Did I need evidence that I was a celiac? Did I care if I wasn't? Was I actually hurting myself by avoiding grains? What would happen if I didn't have enough fiber in my diet? Why was I unable to present my questions in a way to get someone to listen and help me?!

I needed to know what was causing my symptoms, and how to avoid gluten entirely. I needed to know if I should eat chicken and eggs, drink coffee, eat canned tuna. I knew that I felt better when I didn't eat gluten, and I felt terrible when I did. Didn't that mean something?

With time to think came the realization that I didn't want to reintroduce gluten to then be told to eliminate gluten, or possibly to be told to continue eating it. Maybe there was a really good reason for testing, but I didn't know what it was. I was becoming very concerned that I was making a big mistake by not following medical advice, but nothing I was being told to do made any sense to me.

But who was I to go against the directives of expert after expert? I wasn't a trained physician. My health decisions were guided only by my personal experience. The unwavering conviction of every physician I consulted was in direct conflict with my chosen path, and it was deeply troubling.

My decision against the endoscopy led me to another dead end. I briefly considered visiting other doctors in the fields I had previously identified. Maybe a single doctor didn't represent the entire field, and I thought the specialties I picked were good ones, but I didn't move immediately in that direction. I was busy at work and home trying to make up for years of neglect, and I was feeling mentally exhausted. Besides, I felt pretty good physically. I was still taking pain medicine and anti-inflammatories, but hadn't experienced any episodes of extreme pain or exhaustion for a while. I was even experimenting with taking ADD medications as needed rather than routinely.

Just as I was comfortably ignoring the need to address questions about my diet, my knee popped as I ran up a set of stairs and I was unable to walk without support. I went to the emergency room and told my gluten story to the physician treating me because he innocently asked about my health history, completely unaware that he was opening the gates for me to share my medical challenges from the previous thirty years as well as enabling me to try out my newly formed thoughts about the role of food in health.

"Yeah," he said matter-of-factly, "I always talk to my chronic pain patients about food. It's the foundation of health. Not just eating healthy foods and avoiding junk, but figuring out what foods are best and harmful for each individual person."

Whoa. What?? Was I having this conversation?

"Do you think gluten can be causing my problems?" I asked. "Can I resolve them if I figure out what to eat?"

"Absolutely," he said. "Most doctors don't learn about food, but you need to find one who did."

Then he was gone, the demands of a busy emergency room calling him.

I couldn't get all the information I wanted, but I left with a brace on my knee, renewed energy to continue my quest, and restored confidence that I was on the right path.

I thought a lot about what the emergency room physician said, that most doctors don't learn about food. That seemed strange to me. When I was initially researching celiac disease I found that doctors two thousand years ago were very aware of the role of food in health and routinely altered patients' diets to address maladies. Hippocrates, the father of medicine, taught that all illness has a natural cause and was quoted as saying, "Let food be thy medicine and medicine be thy food."

When did medical education and practice stop considering the role of food in disease? Of course, "bad food" such as sugar and trans fat is addressed when it is associated with conditions such as diabetes and heart disease. But it seemed that in the past a

person's diet was examined and adjusted before any other intervention. When did that stop, and why did we start treating symptoms before understanding their cause?

I tried to think through the daily life of a rheumatologist, an
orthopedist, or a general practitioner. If they weren't taught to
think about food, why would they? Nothing in their daily experience would lead them in that direction. They are experts at
diagnosing and treating disease. Representatives selling the latest
drugs, equipment, and technology are literally knocking on their
doors every day to provide free samples and free training. Who
knocks on their door to talk about food?

An orthopedist's job is to repair damage, right? It's not to figure
out what caused damage and stop it from happening. Why would
he be focused on preventing patients from coming to his office? It's
someone else's job to figure out what causes joint inflammation
and damage. But whose job is it?

I thought about the patient's perspective too. Patients go to
a doctor to fix a problem. We are conditioned to expect a quick
solution - a miracle drug or procedure to return us to a function-
ing state. Most patients would probably look for another doctor if
one told them to change their diet rather replacing a bad knee or
instead of giving them a medication to treat their disease.

And maybe I would have looked for a new doctor too, at first. I
was reminded of developing a sinus infection once when I was on
vacation. For years I developed a sinus infection every four to six
months, and was always treated with an antibiotic. Because I was
on vacation, though, I could not see my regular physician. The only
doctor available would not prescribe antibiotics but instead told
me to use a sinus flush, explaining that almost all sinus infectious
clear up on their own in days.

I was furious! I wanted a quick and easy resolution and was
not at all interested in his philosophy about the overprescribing
of antibiotics or their effects on my body. Flushing was gross, and

my vacation was ruined.

Reflecting on my strong feelings with that experience, I imagined that other people would probably react the same way if they didn't receive the treatment they knew was available and would solve their problem. But after years of quick solutions, of medications and surgeries and uncontrolled, dramatically declining health, I think I would have been open to a new approach.

I pondered who would be the appropriate advocate for investigating the cause of certain chronic health problems. I couldn't imagine who would have the incentive to drive this approach and would benefit from the effort. Maybe insurance companies? They required medical imaging to confirm necessity and more conservative attempts for treatment, such as physical therapy and cortisone injections, before authorizing payment for joint surgery. What if a change in diet was required before starting a medication for attention deficit disorder, for example, or prior to prescribing an immunosuppressant? Or maybe before authorizing the sixth joint surgery or approving a second year of medication for chronic pain for patients under the age of forty?

I knew none of this would be popular with patients or physicians and likely not even possible with the challenge of monitoring compliance. I just toyed with the idea, realizing that no other industry would more directly benefit or likely have the ability to cause this type of change.

If I had altered my diet sooner, the companies providing medical insurance for me would have saved hundreds of thousands of dollars on appointments, testing, medication, equipment, and procedures over a thirty-year period.

Chapter Sixteen

NEW WORLD

When I began to experience pain and weakness more frequently, I decided to renew my search for help. The emergency room physician was proof that doctors who knew about food did exist, and he was confident that there were others like him.

At first I found only the same types of physicians I had seen before, but finally I discovered something different. It started with a website explaining that "conventional" or "traditional" medicine is focused on acute care, which is effective in treating injuries and short-term illnesses, but poorly designed to treat the chronic diseases affecting a large portion of the patients physicians see every day. The only remedy conventional doctors have to treat the more than one hundred million Americans who suffer from chronic conditions is a prescription pad for medication intended to suppress or mask symptoms.

Wow. It was very strange to see the only medical approach I'd ever known neatly packaged up and labeled with its flaws so boldly listed. I'd never seen what I considered to be standard medical practice challenged like that. But the assessment made perfect sense to me. The doctors I had been going to didn't know how to help me, other than with medication. But the website promised another way.

A group of physicians recognized that conventional medical practice did not meet the needs of their patient population and designed a better plan called functional medicine. The nonconventional approach was specifically designed to use sophisticated diagnostic methods to determine why disease exists and then design treatment based on each individual's unique combination of genetics, medical history, and lifestyle. Chronic conditions were viewed as preventable and reversible by functional medicine practitioners.

Okay, that sounded perfect. Exactly what I needed. So why wasn't I excited to learn that there were doctors who would very likely accept my story and help me figure out how to solve my problems?

I think because it was hard for me to believe it was true. Who were these doctors, and why hadn't I heard anything about them before? If functional medicine was the solution for millions of patients, wouldn't I have seen an advertisement or known someone who was helped by a functional medicine doctor?

Maybe there was only one guy practicing this kind of medicine, or maybe the approach wasn't scientifically sound. I needed to learn more.

I searched for "functional medicine" to see if there was any additional information. Page after page after page of results returned. Every link I clicked led me to a website built on the same theme of differences between conventional and functional medicine, and an explanation of how functional medicine was the answer for patients suffering with chronic disease. Each was loaded with testimonials from patients who had been restored to health through functional medicine after years of pain and suffering.

Growing optimistic that my frustrations with what I was beginning to think of as "conventional" medicine were valid and could be addressed, I entered the Institute for Functional Medicine website and searched for a physician. I found one a few miles away and requested an appointment.

I wrote:

*I have autoimmune symptoms and blood test results.
I feel much better on a gluten-free diet, but I am still
missing something. I've had no luck with conventional
medicine. I need help figuring out what I can eat, and
what I can do to feel like myself again.*

The next morning I received an email from the doctor asking
if I was available to talk by phone. She said she wanted to get
some additional information before scheduling an appointment.
I chose the first time slot she suggested, at nine thirty that morning, excited about this new direction and curious about what she
wanted to know. My first meeting with a doctor had always been
in the exam room. I couldn't imagine why we needed to talk before
meeting.

I was at work, but found an empty conference room and waited
for her call. The phone rang exactly on time.

"Hello?"

"Hi Ms. McGuire! Thank you for reaching out to me. Can you
tell me what's going on and what led you to me?"

Her voice was warm and calm. I shared my story and responded
to her questions about my goals and concerns. She didn't challenge me or try to explain away anything I said. She didn't even
seem surprised or offended when I told her about my hesitancy to
accept the claims of functional medicine. She simply agreed that
the approach was different than most people were used to, and
shared her ordeal of becoming sick herself and failing to recover
with traditional treatment. Through her illness she recognized the
failings of traditional medicine and discovered functional medicine, which saved her life. Inspired by her experience, she left her
well-established medical practice and entered a program to become
a functional medicine practitioner.

The doctor thanked me for my time and said she looked forward to working with me. The next step was for me to fill out some forms and return them to her with any recent blood test results.

Okay, it was a good start! Nothing seemed unusual except that I spent half an hour talking on the phone with a doctor so she could better understand me and what I was trying to accomplish. I was still afraid I would be disappointed again, but was growing more excited that I might actually be able to finally get all my questions answered about how food was affecting my body.

I'd filled out new-patient forms many times before, so I knew what to expect. Or I thought I did until I started working through her sixteen-page document that evening. The medical history part was familiar enough, so I completed that section first, listing my medications and transferring information about surgeries from a list I prepared once I could no longer recall them all from memory.

I flipped through the rest of the document and found typical questions about diseases that ran in my family, alcohol/tobacco/drug use, and frequency of exercise. Less typically, there were detailed sections related to my childhood, diet, and relationships. Feeling a little overwhelmed by the amount of information requested, I returned to the first page of the form and started working through one section at a time, beginning with a description of my highest-priority issues and success of previous treatments. Easy. Pain and fatigue, gluten-free diet and anti-inflammatories, moderate success.

The questions in the next section focused on exposure to abuse and violence as a child. I balked a little, hoping we weren't going down the "symptoms caused by stress" path my primary care doctor had taken me down before, which resulted in a dead end. I really had no idea how much of an impact childhood stress could have on an adult, but I hoped we could address the food issues clearly affecting my body before analyzing my childhood.

I scanned the form again, realizing that the majority of sections addressed aspects of my life that I never really thought about, much less discussed with a physician. There were questions about my birth, how long I was breast-fed, major changes in my life, how I felt during different seasons of the year, my level of satisfaction with people around me, the number of fillings in my teeth, and the frequency and appearance of bowel movements. While I reasoned that all of it must have been important or it wouldn't have been included on the form, it was unusual enough to trigger doubt and spark defensive thoughts. I began to tell myself that this was not going to be what I was looking for, that I was going to be disappointed, that it was too weird.

But wait. I wanted something different, right? I acknowledged that functional medicine was proudly "nonconventional" and promised to assess and treat the "whole patient" rather than a disease or a symptom. Since that was what drew me to this approach in the first place, I should just trust the process and march on. What else was I going to do? I certainly wasn't going to give up because the new-patient forms were a little odd. I expected treatment to be different, so why did I expect the intake process to be the same as that used by physicians who had not been able to help me?

I smiled a little as I realized my reluctance to let go of the old process that was comfortable and familiar, but a piece of medical practices that had not been right for me for years.

Working my way through the document, I was encouraged by a five-page section with more than 250 symptoms to review. I selected dozens that applied to me, including many that seemed meaningful because they worsened as my pain and fatigue grew. Those specific symptoms, such as cold hands and feet, pale skin, cracked skin on hands, and mouth sores, had been completely ignored or immediately dismissed as meaningless by every previous doctor.

The section on diet was also inspiring and filled me with hope and curiosity, since the number and depth of the questions seemed to indicate that food was also a critical component of my health history. It probed food cravings and aversions as well as how much of very specific food and drink items I consumed and how they made me feel as a child and as an adult.

I was anxious to see how all the seemingly unrelated pieces of information would come together and how the doctor would use that information to move forward. I returned the completed form with renewed enthusiasm, along with the blood test results from my primary care physician and the doctor who performed allergy testing.

The doctor reviewed my medical history and test results, then sent an email asking for authorization to order additional tests to help determine what was causing my symptoms and the problems with my immune system. I agreed, and she said the testing facilities would send testing kits directly to me by mail.

I arrived home from work three days later to find one large envelope in the mailbox and two small cardboard boxes on the porch from three different testing laboratories. I took them into the house and opened them immediately on the kitchen island. Chris and Kenny abandoned their homework and joined me as I removed the contents of each package.

I didn't know what to expect, since the biggest role I'd ever played in testing was to show up at the lab with an order for a blood draw, and even that was unusual because my blood was usually drawn at the doctor's office. As I watched Kenny inspect a lancet apparently used to obtain a blood sample while Chris played with a disposable pipette from one of the boxes, I realized this was very much a do-it-yourself affair. Each kit came with a set of instructions and supplies needed for sample collection.

When the boys lost interest and returned to their homework, I put the materials back in their original packages to keep from mixing them up. I was a little overwhelmed by my apparent role in the process, but wanted to get started right away so I could learn more about what was going on with my body and get closer to a solution.

I started with the envelope because it had fewer components and seemed less intimidating than the two boxes filled with tubes. I unfolded the double-sided requisition form and found that the doctor selected "IgG food allergy" from the long list of tests available. After I completed a section about insurance, the form directed me to a website to determine the amount of payment I should submit. I plopped down at the table between the boys with my laptop.

My insurance company did not have a contract with the testing laboratory, and the IgG test was not excluded for coverage (it was complicated), so I was responsible for 20 percent of the test cost. I checked a price list, did the math, and wrote a check. At the end of the form I provided information for research purposes about my symptoms and conditions, then folded it back up with my payment tucked inside.

Out of curiosity, I clicked around before leaving the testing laboratory website. The company described itself as a world leader in diagnostic testing for chronic disease. It offered panels of tests for conditions such as attention deficit disorder, chronic fatigue, and fibromyalgia, and provided free resources for patients and physicians. Blogs, articles, and webinars examined the latest research on topics such as the role of food and supplements in treating autism, the connection between chronic inflammation and disease, the role of gut bacteria in health, and the relationship between heavy metals and psychiatric disorders. The website advertised a number of events, including workshops hosted by the laboratory as well as functional medicine conferences held all over the world.

Wow! This do-it-yourself kit was not assembled in someone's garage, as I had imagined when I first dumped what looked like middle school science supplies onto my island. It seemed to be a well-researched analytical tool created by a professional organization that was connected to the larger functional medicine community.

I checked the websites for the other two testing laboratories and was awed by the scope of available testing, the existence of huge amounts of scientific research related to chronic disease, and the functional medicine community's apparent comfort with addressing difficult medical issues.

I wanted to be enthusiastic about the wealth of information available through functional medicine, which seemed logical and scientifically based, but I continued to struggle with an inability to explain why I had never heard about it before and why so many good doctors were not using it or talking about it. Nobody ever mentioned any of these tests or referred me to a functional medicine doctor for help with my chronic health problems. Why was there such a discrepancy in testing and treatment methods between traditional and functional medicine? The functional medicine community was clearly different, but was their approach valid?

I decided to just complete the testing. I would follow the process and then I could determine for myself whether functional medicine worked to improve my health.

The IgG food allergy test required a blood sample. I filled five dime-sized circles on a thick paper card with blood from my finger. Once dry I would simply drop the card into the overnight shipping bag provided, add the requisition form and payment, then ship it to the lab. That was pretty easy!

Growing more confident in my at-home sampling abilities, I opened the instructions inside one of the boxes for a "comprehensive GI profile." It was a stool sample kit. I was to collect a specimen and transfer samples to each of the collection tubes.

Well, okay. This one could wait.

The final test was similar to the stool sample kit, except the tubes were for blood. My job was to fill out the form, label the tubes, then go to a blood draw center for collection. I made an appointment online at the closest location, which turned out to be an urgent care facility.

When I arrived with my kit a couple of days later, the waiting room was bustling with sick children, injured teens, and construction workers in hard hats and muddy boots waiting for routine drug tests. Nobody else held a cardboard box like mine. When my name was called, the nurse led me to a room where she expertly unpacked and organized the contents of the box on the exam table. She drew my blood, checked a few boxes and signed a few lines on the form, repacked everything, wrapped one rubber band around the top of the box and another around the sides, dropped the box into the shipping bag, slapped on the prepaid label, then thanked me and wished me a good day.

The urgent care clinic was just one of many collection sites in my area, and the nurse I met was just one of many at the clinic. Even if she was the clinic's expert in this testing, surely others must have known the process. So how many people were getting this type of testing done, and who was ordering the tests? Was it all through functional medicine physicians? How big was this system?

Functional medicine was beginning to feel like a huge secret movement operating in plain sight.

Chapter Seventeen

FUNCTIONAL SOLUTION

A couple of weeks after completing the sample collections, the doctor was ready to meet. I was so excited to finally get all my questions answered, and eager to find out how functional medicine methods would be used to help me.

The doctor's office was in a plain two-story professional building, the sign for her practice sandwiched between those of an insurance agent and a military recruiter. The tan brick structure looked like it was probably built in the 1950s. It was very boxy, with square windows and black metal railing along the three concrete steps to the external door of each office.

I opened the door under her office number and entered a narrow space with a small retrofitted elevator on the right and a dark set of stairs to the back left. I climbed the stairs and stepped into a bright hallway with brass light fixtures and colorful prints along both walls. The pale gray paint looked fresh, and the gold pattern in the navy blue carpet was very classy.

The doctor's name was printed on a door at the end of the hall. I went in, and felt like I had just walked into someone's family room. Couches and matching chairs faced a large coffee table in the middle of the room, and short bookshelves filled with toys and books lined the walls. The only indication of a medical practice was a stand of brochures on one of the bookshelves providing information about health conditions and services offered. A hallway led off the back of the room to a series of closed doors. I didn't hear or see anyone, so I took a seat on a couch.

I was trying to identify an action figure sticking out of a toy bin across the room when a tall woman in flowing dark slacks and a cream-colored blouse entered from the hallway. She moved with the grace of an athlete, the slight inward curl at the end of her shoulder-length brown hair bouncing a little with each long stride as she approached me with her hand outstretched.

"Hi!" she said as she took my hand in both of hers. "It's great to finally meet you!"

She led me down the hallway to her office at the end, taking a quick detour into a kitchen along the way to get us both a bottle of water.

Sunlight streamed into her office from a slim window, dividing the room in half. In the office half to the right, a black easy chair faced a small desk holding a laptop and a stack of papers. In the clinical side to the left a large plant stood at the head of a thickly padded exam table covered by a cotton sheet and a soft blanket.

The doctor said she wanted to perform a brief exam and asked me to climb onto the table. While I appreciated the cozy atmosphere, the experience felt a little odd without the cold, hard exam table and crinkly paper I knew so well.

The doctor took my blood pressure, listened to my heart and lungs, pushed on my stomach, and looked at my knuckles. She said she was checking for inflammation and joint damage. I had some, but no more than she expected.

For the next hour I sat in the easy chair across from her at the desk, listened carefully, and took notes as she reviewed the new patient information I provided and every test result in detail. She discussed the reason for each question and sample analysis, and shared her thoughts on the relevance of the response or outcome.

Finally, she looked up at me from her stack of papers.

"A combination of your genetics, environment, and lifestyle resulted in autoimmune activity that is damaging your joints and thyroid, as well as affecting your energy and focus. You are genetically predisposed to autoimmune disease, and factors from the day you were born, such as breast-feeding, infections, use of antibiotics, food choices, and stress have altered the function of your immune system and led to the expression of your health problems."

Her tone was grave as she pointed out the presence of multiple food allergies, an unhealthy balance of gut bacteria, and a global infection identified in my test results, which indicated that my immune system was under significant strain and was struggling to function effectively.

"You are now at a critical juncture," she said. "Your condition will continue to deteriorate and you will express additional symptoms and disease if you do not repair your immune system."

Feeling thoroughly defeated, I slid slowly down in my seat, waiting for her to gently tell me I was the worst case she had ever seen and that my situation was hopeless.

Instead, she smiled.

"We need to fix your leaky gut, remove your toxins, address your nutrient deficiencies, and balance your gut biome."

I really didn't understand what any of that meant, but her matter-of-fact presentation and obvious confidence in our ability to do those things made me feel better.

I straightened in my chair. "So you have seen something like this before?"

She gave me a worn expression I didn't comprehend. "Every day."

She must have noticed the expectant look on my face because she flipped over a page of my test results and started to draw.

"Leaky gut is a key issue you need to resolve to get your health under control," she said.

She drew a squiggly line with what looked like rocks lined tightly beneath.

"This is how the intestinal lining should look, with very little open space. These spaces are really small pores between the cells, which allow minerals and nutrients to pass through into the bloodstream."

She then drew rocks spaced far apart.

"The pores are sometimes opened too much, and things that should be blocked can get through the larger openings. Undigested food, bacteria, and toxins should stay in the gut but pass through the bigger holes into the bloodstream, causing all kinds of problems, including food allergies, because the immune system reacts to food that shouldn't be found moving through the body outside the digestive system."

She put down her pen and looked at me earnestly.

"Leaky gut is thought to be very common, affecting millions of people. It is a very serious problem that can and should be addressed. It can be caused by too much sugar in the diet, because eating too much sugar can lead to high levels of yeast, which increases the size of the pores. It can also be caused by some medicines such as nonsteroidal anti-inflammatories that are known to damage the intestinal lining, allowing larger particles that should be blocked to go through. Also, too much bad bacteria in the gut, stress, and excessive alcohol consumption can increase intestinal permeability."

There was stress again. Maybe I flinched or maybe she was used to patients questioning the effects of stress, because she immediately clarified. "Stress can be not only mental, but also physical from too much exercise, too little sleep, or consuming substances that cause an undesirable response, which is highly individual, but could include sensitivities to specific foods, drinks, or medication."

I assumed she would tell me later what I was supposed to do about my sugar addiction, damaging medications, and bad gut bacteria. I bulleted the three items under a heading "fix leaky gut" in my notes and added a star reminding me to come back to it later.

"Gluten," she said, "is a major cause of leaky gut. Not only does it cause intestinal irritation and inflammation because it is difficult to digest, it also increases the amount of a protein called zonulin that widens the pores in the intestinal lining."

She stopped and allowed me to catch up in my note taking. "Leaky gut is closely connected to autoimmune disease because the continuous reaction of the immune system to foreign particles in the bloodstream leads to a stressed and less accurate immune system that sometimes begins attacking the body's own cells. The immune system creates antibodies for the foreign particles in the bloodstream, and some of those particles - gluten and dairy in particular - are very similar to tissues in the body, which get attacked by mistake and results in a long list of symptoms in addition to food allergies and sensitivities. Joint pain, skin conditions, sore muscles, chronic infections, seasonal allergies, fatigue, anxiety, and brain fog, as well as advanced autoimmune disease. Your autoimmune condition will continue to progress and you will likely be diagnosed with additional autoimmune diseases if you don't fix your leaky gut."

She slid the stack of test results across her desk to me and returned to her own notes to review our plan. The first step was a detoxification diet to rid my body of substances causing inflammation and to heal my gut. She gave me a single-page flyer highlighting a six-week program I could order online. The program would provide very specific information about what to eat and would supply a number of nutritional supplements to rotate over the six-week period.

In general, during detox I was to avoid eggs, dairy, soy, coffee, caffeine, grains, gluten, white potatoes, peppers, eggplant, beans, nuts, seeds, sugar, alcohol, and processed food. I should limit my carbohydrate intake to less than fifty grams per day. The diet allowed most vegetables and meats, fermented foods, specific low glycemic fruits, coconut, and many spices.

As the doctor circled a website for more information about the detox program, I suddenly realized that I had not yet received a clear answer to my most basic question.

"Am I a celiac?" I asked.

"Well, I think so," she said. "Based on your history and test results I think it is very likely."

She flipped through the stack of papers in front of me and highlighted a few test results that supported her opinion. She said there were other tests she could perform, but the only truly conclusive test was an endoscopy, to look at damage to the small intestine when gluten is being consumed regularly. After further discussion and a second, more cursory review of my immunology results showing high levels of autoimmune activity, we agreed that our immediate focus should be toward restoring my health rather than a firm diagnosis.

For the last part of our appointment, as we transitioned from an explanation of what was going on with me to actions to take, I could no longer process the volume of new information and switched from involved participation to silent note taking. She hit upon a number of clearly important topics, and I did my best to capture the information.

I left with a mixture of information and directives to sort through later.

- It would take six months to a year for my leaky gut to heal.
- My damaged joints and thyroid could not be healed, but fixing my immune system would prevent further damage. Body aches, brain fog, and tiredness would go away.
- Lectins are proteins in some plants that can cause digestive issues. They may be a plant defense to prevent being eaten. Beans and nuts are high in lectins. I should avoid high-lectin foods so my gut

would heal. Lentils are okay. After detox I could try
pumpkin and sunflower seeds.

- Two thirds of the immune system lives in the gut.
- It takes months to recover from the effects of a single exposure to gluten.
- Soy can act like hormones in the human body. I
should avoid soy.
- Improving my gut biome helps with leaky gut. My gut
biome was probably affected by many ear infections
and antibiotics in my childhood. The bacteria in the
gut has a huge impact on human health. I should
take probiotics and eat foods that feed good bacteria.
- GMO corn might be affecting our gut biome. It was
banned in the European Union and in Mexico. I
should try to avoid GMO foods while healing my gut.
- I was likely suffering from adrenal fatigue, a condition where my adrenal gland was overstimulated
and unable to keep up with demand, contributing to
my brain fog and tiredness. Eliminating caffeine and
ADD medications, as well as taking a supplement for
adrenal support, should help restore function.
- She recommended several supplements, including
fish oil as well as thyroid and adrenal support, plus
a number of natural remedies for inflammation and
pain relief. They were available through a high-qual-
ity manufacturer whose ingredients she trusted, or I
could get them at a vitamins shop. She would send a
link to the manufacturer's website, plus her physician code for a discount.
- Watch personal hygiene products for gluten. I
should select items such as toothpaste, shampoo, lip
balm, soap, deodorant, hair dye, and lotion that do
not contain gluten.

- Since I still frequently suffered from mouth sores, I should buy a toothpaste without lauryl sulfate. Lauryl sulfate could be an irritant, and was an ingredient in the brand I used. She suggested a few brands I'd never heard of.
- Chronic inflammation caused by food allergies and sensitivities, toxins, chronic infections (Lyme disease, yeast, molds, etc.), and stress leads to cancer and other diseases.
- I should follow the "dirty dozen" and "clean thirteen" guidance when shopping for produce. It's an annual ranking of popular fruits and vegetables by level of pesticide contamination. I should buy organic for the highest-ranking items (the dirty dozen), but could safely buy nonorganic for those found to have the lowest levels (the clean thirteen).
- I should check out organic markets where I could more easily find healthy products. She recommended a few local ones.
- For my knee pain, the joint that was bothering the most at the time, I should consider platelet-rich plasma therapy, where my own platelets could be injected to help heal joint damage. She would send me a link for more information.
- Don't lick envelopes. The glue can contain gluten.
- Acupuncturists and neurostimulators could help with my back pain as I eliminated anti-inflammatory and painkilling drugs. She would send a link.
- My dosage of thyroid medication was not sufficient. She would send a prescription for a natural brand to my pharmacy.
- I should get to know my local farmers so I could find out what they feed their animals. If they are fed

grain, I might have a reaction when I eat the meat. I could find grass-fed beef at most grocery stores, but I needed to ask farmers about poultry.

- She provided several references to research zonulin, the protein that widens gaps in the intestinal lining when gluten is consumed. There was a lot of relevant and interesting research in this area.
- When I drink alcohol, it should come from grapes only (not grains).
- Because I had a number of mercury fillings in my teeth, I should consider consulting with a functional dentist. The fillings may cause increased levels of mercury in my body, but exposure can be much higher if they are removed improperly.
- My iodine levels were extremely low and needed supplementation. I should buy salt with no iodine so I can better control my levels. Sea salt is good.
- Nightshades such as tomatoes, bell peppers, and eggplant cause arthritis flares.
- During detox I should eat every three to four hours, and eat nothing after 7:00 p.m.
- I would be billed $775 through PayPal for my first appointment. Future visits would be shorter and less expensive. I would receive an itemized bill that I could submit to insurance. They may reimburse some portion of the cost. Supplements were not likely covered by insurance, but my prescription for thyroid medicine would be.
- I would receive an email follow-up to our visit with links and other important information.

The doctor stood and thanked me for my time, saying she looked forward to our journey together. She gave me a warm hug and said she was always available if I needed her.

For a moment I just stared at her, feeling like a naïve and unprepared little kid suddenly abandoned by my caregiver in a big adult world I didn't begin to understand. I picked up the large stack of test results and notes, forced a weak smile, and walked out of the office.

Behind the wheel of my car I looked at the dozens of pages in my lap, feeling too overwhelmed to leave. How would I even begin to address all the things in my life that were wrong? I sat for a long time in limbo, not wanting to drive away from such an amazing resource that had been so difficult to find, someone clearly capable of unraveling the pieces of complex information that were critical to my health.

I wished I could follow this doctor around with a notepad for months, asking questions and absorbing her knowledge. To start, I wanted to understand how bacteria could be good and corn could be bad, where natural thyroid medicine came from, if I should have the fillings pulled out of my teeth, what PayPal was, why gluten might be in my shampoo, what organic meant, and how I could get to know my local farmers.

Finally motivated by a concern that the doctor would see me sitting in the parking lot and think something was wrong with me, I began the drive home. I promised myself that I would return to my thoughts and notes when I could take the time needed to get organized, then tried to clear my mind and think about something else. It was late afternoon and I wasn't planning to return to work, so I would have time to prepare a nice dinner.

What should we have for dinner? That simple challenge came with a sense of panic, then crushing defeat as I realized that once again I had no idea what I should or shouldn't eat. Should I start the limitations we discussed right away, or wait for the detox diet? It didn't make sense to continue eating things that she said I should avoid. What were those new restrictions?

I remembered jotting down no GMO or high-lectin foods such

as beans and nuts, no corn, no soy. Did she say no potatoes? Why was that? What about all the foods I was sensitive to?

I could clearly picture the colorful pages of food allergy test results, with specific foods listed down the left side of the page and a black bar indicating my reaction to each stretching out to the right. The bar moved through a scale from green, then yellow and orange, and possibly into red, depending on the degree of the response. A number of the foods I ate regularly ended in orange, and several in red, indicating a very strong reaction.

Should I avoid those now too? Why would I eat them if they were causing inflammation in my body? She said chronic inflammation caused, what, cancer? I certainly wanted to avoid that if possible. Eggs and dairy showed very strong results. And yeast? Was that the kind of yeast in bread? And no GMOs. What did that mean? What kinds of food had GMOs?

Ugh. How was I going to figure everything out? Why didn't I ask her what I could eat?!

Chapter Eighteen

TRANSITION

At a traffic light I reached into my pocket and pulled out several white tablets. I broke a pain pill in half and tossed it in my mouth, then bit off a chunk of caffeine and swallowed them without water. I was no longer affected by the bitter taste. The pain in my back had been escalating since early in the doctor's visit. Caffeine seemed to make pain medicine more effective, so I hoped the combination would lessen my discomfort.

I was anxious to get out of the car and hopeful that I could find something to eat. I took a short detour to one of the organic markets the doctor told me about. I had passed it many times but never paid any attention to it. It was small and quietly tucked in with a strip of other shops.

I entered into a small produce area and had the sense of walking into a warehouse because of the wide aisles and plain concrete floors. But then I noticed the brightly colored fruit and vegetables in neatly organized displays with little handwritten signs, which felt warm and welcoming. A huge sign hanging from the ceiling announced that all produce was certified organic, and another explained that the produce section was small because freshness is more important than volume.

Everything in the produce area was organic? Fantastic!

I picked up a sweet potato and turned it over in my hand,

thinking I would have no way to know it was organic without the sign. It didn't look any different, but a little smaller than normal, maybe. As I watched a lady next to me place about half a dozen long, incredibly orange carrots with leaves and roots still attached directly into her cart, I realized that most of the produce was not packaged. I was used to seeing heaps of bagged oranges, apples, onions, and potatoes at my store, but here almost everything was loosely stacked or piled into a crate. Bags were available for customers to use just like any other produce section, but they were made from recycled material and people didn't seem to be using them. I put the sweet potato in my cart, and moved on to explore the rest of the store.

My entire life I had only shopped in big chain grocery stores and was quickly realizing that this one was very different. For one thing, there were signs everywhere. Not signs advertising a product or trumpeting a sales price, but providing information about a group of products or introducing a supplier. Towering over the refrigerated section were beautiful photos of farmers with their products, including one from Maryland who sourced milk.

Out of curiosity, I looked below his photo into the cooler and found glass bottles of milk from a number of farms, each with the farm name prominently printed on the label. The bottles from one farm contained raw milk from grass-fed cows. Interesting! What was raw milk? Did I usually drink cooked milk? Too bad dairy was off my list and I couldn't try it.

As I moved through the store I was aware that I didn't recognize any product labels. And, actually, I didn't recognize a number of the products! I stopped in front of a large section of seaweed snacks. I'd never heard of anyone eating seaweed. Was it a popular snack? As I inspected a large package of seaweed, uhm, slices, I noticed a little "verified non-GMO" label at the bottom right corner. A number of other packages had the same label. I had never seen it before. I wondered if products at my regular grocery store had that label, or if I could only get non-GMO products at an organic market. At least I knew where to find them.

After I saw the non-GMO label the first time, I saw it everywhere. The huge section of chips was covered with it. When I looked closer, I saw that the chips were not made of corn or potato, but of things such as cauliflower, beets, and Brussels sprouts.

I picked up a bag and read the label, wondering what a cauliflower chip would taste like. I returned the chips and moved on to a huge section of cereals, where off-brand varieties boasted ingredients such as amaranth, buckwheat, spelt, millet, kamut, and sprouted corn. Sprouted corn? What's sprouted corn?

I was drawn to a drab section of paper products because they were so different from the festive display of picnic cups, plates, and plastic forks and spoons I was used to. Here the paper towels, napkins, toilet paper, and paper plates were made from recycled material, and some were brown because they were made from unbleached paper. Spoons were made of plant starch, and there were reusable bamboo straws. All the cleaning products were eco-friendly.

They certainly were serious about protecting and restoring the environment through their commitment to reducing waste (of course I saw this on a sign).

It hit me as I stood numbly in front of a sign that said "grind your own nut butter" that I was completely out of my league. I had no idea what nut butter was or what it was used for, and was unprepared to purchase any anyway because I didn't bring my own container from home, like the people around me examining labels on the bulk containers of nuts.

I wondered how obvious it was that I didn't belong. Nobody seemed to pay any attention to me standing around watching them, reading labels, and pushing a lone sweet potato around the store in my cart. Maybe they were used to lost souls wandering in from a different world, curious about another way. Did the wanderers come back? How did the people grinding nut butter get here?

Passing through the coffee section, I noticed a sign that said the coffee was fair wage, shade grown, and direct trade. It was roasted in the store, and the roast date was written on the bin. I truly respected the consistency of the humanitarian and environmental efforts as I moved on to investigate school supplies that included reusable sandwich bags, pens made of bamboo instead of plastic, and journals printed on recycled paper. There were even organic clothes! The sign said the clothes were made without chemicals, with reduced greenhouse emissions, and no child labor. The bug repellent at the end of the aisle was even natural/plant based, made of lemon and eucalyptus.

Could the people in this store be the smartest people in the world? Was everyone in the large groceries using store-provided containers for their bulk purchases, buying chips made of potatoes and milk in plastic jugs just completely clueless about the error of their ways? If the organic market movement was right on, shouldn't it have been more popular?

I looked at the single sweet potato in my cart and suddenly wondered if it was included in the potato ban. I typed "is a sweet potato a potato" on my phone and learned that sweet potatoes are root vegetables and not tubers like a regular potato. But they are tuberous roots.

My shoulders dropped and I sighed out loud. I didn't know if I could eat root vegetables or tuber roots. How could eating be so difficult?

As I turned to go to the front of the store to return the potato, I noticed a section of toothpaste next to unwrapped soap bars made of goat's milk. Thinking the trip wouldn't be completely wasted if I could find gluten-free toothpaste, I picked up a tube and read the label. No indication whether it was gluten-free, but it did have activated charcoal and apparently intentionally did not include fluoride. Why would toothpaste boast the exclusion of fluoride?

Would I ever understand all of this?

I put the toothpaste back and returned to the front of the store, plopping the potato back in its crate on my way out the door.

I didn't find a single thing I could eat. All the items in the massive gluten-free area were made of grains and/or nuts, and there was soy in almost everything. Frozen dinners had wheat, rice, soy, yeast, potatoes, or tomatoes. Even the sausage I found had rice and potatoes. The chips contained yeast and a grain called sorghum. I considered buying a carton of blueberries when I returned the potato, but they hardly seemed worth what felt like a monumental effort required to figure out the unfamiliar checkout process and face the peppy cashiers.

I drove home tired and hungry. Not knowing what I would eat next made me feel like I was starving. And my back was killing me. I swallowed the remaining half of the pain pill from my pocket, and another chunk of caffeine. Where was I going to find something I could eat?

I blasted the radio and shut out all other thoughts.

Once I got home, I immediately slipped off my shoes and gingerly lowered myself to the floor in the living room. Flat on my back with my feet on the couch, I closed my eyes and enjoyed relief from my cramping muscles for the first time in hours. My stomach grumbled from hunger and too much caffeine.

Within seconds, Chris stood over me and asked about dinner. Knowing he was sensitive to my moods and worried when I was in pain, I forced myself to pause before blurting out an irritated, "Eat whatever you want."

I took a breath and remembered leftover meatloaf and mashed potatoes, Chris's favorites, in the refrigerator. He was happy with the suggestion to heat them up with some canned green beans. I hoped there would be enough left for Kenny.

As Chris busied himself in the kitchen, I wondered again what I was going to eat. Certainly not what Chris was having. Beans and potatoes were out, and I used crackers made of some kind of gluten-free grain in the meatloaf. I would have to look for something else. I rolled over with a groan and awkwardly stood up, my back muscles immediately protesting and nearly dropping me to my knees.

I shuffled to the kitchen cabinets to inspect their contents. There were taco shells and seasoning, but the shells were made of corn and the seasoning had milk and potato starch. Gluten-free pasta was made from rice, and pasta sauce from tomatoes. Sloppy joe sauce was also tomato-based. Peanut butter was not an option because of lectins in the nuts. I couldn't eat the canned beans or corn.

There was canned tuna. I turned it over in my hand, wondering what I could do with it. I couldn't make tuna cheese melts because cheese, gluten-free bread, and mayonnaise were not allowed. Gluten-free bread had rice, eggs, and yeast, and mayonnaise was made with eggs and soy.

Did the doctor say something about avoiding tuna because of high mercury levels? I returned the can to the cabinet and quickly flipped through my notes but couldn't find anything about it. Just acknowledging the stack of papers from the doctor's office made me anxious. Half of me wanted to toss them in the trash and pretend we never met, while the other half wanted to sit down and research every single item until I understood everything.

Forcing myself to reject both options for the moment, I neatly stacked my notes and returned to my food search. There was a pound of ground beef in the refrigerator, but it wasn't grass-fed. At least I didn't think it was. I couldn't find anything on the label indicating what the cows ate. I put the beef back and took a pack of hot dogs out of the crisper. Corn syrup was listed as an ingredient, but I reasoned that maybe corn syrup wasn't exactly corn and there couldn't really be much corn syrup in a hot dog.

I was getting desperate. Was any amount of corn too much?

What did the doctor say was the negative effect of eating corn?

As I considered eating the hot dogs anyway, my eyes fixed on a bottle of orange juice. I stared at it hopefully. The only ingredients were orange juice and orange juice pulp. The juice wasn't organic, but maybe that was okay? I picked up my phone to find out if oranges were one of the dirty dozen or the clean thirteen. My silent chant, "clean thirteen, clean thirteen," was disrupted by learning that the clean list was actually fifteen. I thought that was a good sign. That meant there were two additional fruits or vegetables that didn't have to be organic.

I scanned the updated dirty dozen and clean fifteen lists to find that oranges weren't included at all. What did that mean? Oranges weren't found to have the highest pesticide levels, or lowest either. So should the juice be organic or not? I had no idea. With just a little hesitation, I filled a large glass and drank the juice while I investigated the freezer. No better luck there. My frozen enchiladas were made with beans, corn, cheese, milk, tomatoes, rice, and bell peppers. The gluten-free pizza listed rice, potatoes, peppers, garlic, yeast, and soy on the label.

I was running out of options.

I scanned the pantry shelves filled with snack bars, chips, and cereal, all with ingredients I couldn't eat. I closed the door, then drank another glass of orange juice and ate tuna out of the can. Unwilling to face the usual chore of packing my lunch for the next day, I took another pain pill and went to bed.

After several terribly restless hours of tossing and turning in an attempt to lessen the pain in my irritated back, I finally got up and paced around the house in the dark. No amount of medication helped if I stayed in one position too long, but walking in my tennis shoes with a heat pad on my lower back soothed a little.

My dazed slog back and forth in the living room with heavy feet and half-closed eyes reminded me of comforting the kids in the middle of the night when they were babies. I warmed at the memory of how tiny and dependent they were, such a contrast to the strong individuals they had become. When the room began to lighten with the rising sun, the surreal atmosphere evaporated and my thoughts turned to more practical matters.

I clicked on the television and brewed a pot of coffee. Gazing into my second cup, I wondered how I was going to live without it. During detox I couldn't have caffeine or coffee. How would that work? I didn't think I would be able to function, especially after a night like the one I just had. With a shudder and a slowly growing sense of alarm, I finished my second cup and poured a third.

The coffee made me hungry and irritated. Or maybe hunger made me irritated. My frustrations from the day before returned in full force as I searched for something to eat for breakfast.

I thought finding gluten-free food was difficult, but this was impossible. I was upset not only because I was hungry and didn't know what to eat, but also because I was motivated to eat the right food with no idea how to do that or what my next steps were to figure it out.

In an attempt to calm my growing exasperation, I decided to do the best I could and not to strive for perfection right away. Detox would start in a couple of weeks and I would be told exactly what to eat. Until then I would try not to obsess about every bite I put in my mouth.

Right. Easier said than done. I knew I would struggle to suppress the thought that I was hurting myself with every bite of food from the "avoid" list.

I took the container of orange juice out of the refrigerator, shook it, and immediately drank the remaining half bottle, leaving the empty container by my purse to remind me to buy more. Still feeling disgruntled despite my sincere attempts at optimism, I quickly ran through the list of what I couldn't eat for breakfast.

No bagel with cream cheese, no cereal, no eggs, no toast. What about bacon? The ingredients looked fine to me. I fried up half a package and greedily chomped it down as I considered what to take for lunch.

I was tempted to avoid the subject of lunch entirely by planning to pick something up from one of the many restaurants in the area, but tried to face the issue maturely and admit that I wouldn't be able to find anything then and would be rushed and hungry. With the energy and enthusiasm of a sloth, I once more began the meal evaluation process. I considered and rejected my typical lunch of a peanut butter and jelly sandwich with chips and a gluten-free cookie, since every bit of it was banned.

Was lunch meat okay? I couldn't have bread or mayonnaise, but what about sliced turkey? The package listed cornstarch as an ingredient. I growled out loud.

Forget it. I had to eat something! I was taking the turkey. Just sticking pieces of meat in a plastic bag seemed weird. I'd heard of lettuce wraps as a healthy alternative to bread, and thought that was how I could take my turkey to work.

I examined our container of romaine lettuce, determined it nonorganic, then pulled up the dirty dozen and clean fifteen lists on my phone. Lettuce wasn't on either list. Wouldn't it be the same as other leafy vegetables? Cabbage was listed as clean, spinach as dirty. That didn't really help.

I wrapped my questionable turkey slices in questionable lettuce, grabbed a banana, which also was not on either list, and threw them into my lunch bag.

Done. I didn't want to think any more about it.

Before lunch, I received a long email from the doctor with a summary of what we discussed the afternoon before, references to research, and actions to take. She listed the supplements I needed to get before and after detox, and provided information about how best to contact her during business hours as well as at night and on weekends. She attached the detox program specifics and a detailed bill.

The email didn't address my struggle with food at all, and reminded me of how much I had to do and learn. The amount of information was again overwhelming, but the organized structure of her message was less intimidating than my jumbled pile of notes and gave me perspective about what was most important.

Clearly the emphasis was on detox and supplementation. I decided that would be my focus too, and planned to order the detox kit and buy the prescribed supplements before diving any deeper into the mass of other new topics.

I was surprised by the relief I felt from that small bit of clarity around next steps, and knew I also had to do something to clear up my frustration about food. As I ate my interesting but not really satisfying lettuce-wrapped turkey and the banana, I listed on a legal pad as much as I could remember about what I shouldn't eat and why.

Once I had written everything down, it was pretty obvious that food allergies were the most important category for me to avoid. The rest were important too, but I reasoned that it was not necessary to meet each requirement before starting detox since the program was specifically designed to address everything on the list.

And, of course, avoiding gluten was a high priority.

I smiled at the list I made. No eggs, dairy, yeast, grains, or gluten.

Okay, I could do that! I had no idea if my logic was clinically valid, but it worked for me. The restrictions felt manageable and I would be able to eat food I determined was at a lower priority without too much angst. It was only temporary. Comforted and feeling much more confident, I put away the list and my lunch bag and got back to work.

That evening I received an invoice from PayPal for the new-patient visit and very easily sent payment to the doctor. I knew the price of the first visit before we met, but I had been so focused on the necessity of her help that I didn't think much about it. But I thought quite a bit about it as I charged $775 to my credit card. No doubt her time was worth her rate and I truly believed that my health was dependent on her guidance, but that was a lot of money. And it wasn't the only expense. I had already paid $300 to $400 for each of the three diagnostic kits the doctor ordered prior to the appointment, and the detox program would be $640. No telling how much the additional supplements would cost, and I needed nine of them.

I was by no means financially comfortable, and apparently insurance was not going to cover most of these new expenses. There was also acupuncture, a neurostimulator, platelet injections in my knee, and a functional dentist to consider.

How much would those things cost? Were they essential to my healing? There was no way I would have enough money for everything. I didn't really have funds for what I was already committed to do. I would have to prioritize treatments according to what I could afford.

Chapter Nineteen

DETOX

The next day I didn't have the time or energy to do anything with the information from my visit. Then early Saturday morning I sat down with my laptop and notes, ready to get started.

I felt like I needed to organize all the "to do" items before I took any action and quickly became lost researching topics the doctor mentioned in passing, such as how and why people with thyroid disease should effectively maintain appropriate iodine levels, and the molecular similarities between soy and gluten.

Each search led to multiple additional subjects and questions. While all of the topics were incredibly interesting, I realized I could spend days diving deeper and deeper into one area without any resolution and with no progress toward addressing my priorities.

I put my notes aside, made rough mental "now," "next," and "later" lists to convince myself that I wasn't neglecting important issues, then wrote "detox" and "supplements" on a sticky note with the word "now" at the top. I would worry about the others later.

I ordered the supplements the doctor recommended and the detox kit. A number of documents related to the detox program were attached to the doctor's email, so I clicked through them to get an idea of what it would be like. They included information explaining the goals and approach of the program; a chart detailing the supplements I would take for each phase; a list of foods to eat and foods to avoid; and a sample diet plan with recipes for breakfast, lunch, dinner, and snacks.

I became more excited with every word I read. The detox program was going to help heal my gut and calm my immune system, eliminate chronic inflammation, and help me avoid chronic disease. It was what I had been looking for! I was very anxious to see how good I could feel.

And there was a diet plan! Fantastic! I had to wait for the kit to arrive to officially start detox, but I could start the meals right away. Finally I would know what to eat!!

The program included detox and intestinal healing phases, each with a number of supplements to support those processes. The food restrictions were consistent for the entire program, eliminating foods from my diet that cause intestinal inflammation so I could heal my gut. No grains, dairy, eggs, gluten, soy, nuts, seeds, tomatoes, peppers, mushrooms, sugar, coffee, caffeine, or alcohol.

I could eat most vegetables and fermented foods such as kimchi, kombucha, and pickled sauerkraut. Most meats were allowed, but fish needed to be wild caught, chicken and turkey had to be hormone- and antibiotic-free, bacon uncured, and beef needed to be grass-fed and hormone- and antibiotic-free. Low-glycemic fruits were allowed, as was coconut in pretty much any form (butter, cream, milk, oil, flakes, or yogurt). Lots of herbs and spices were okay, and I should drink herbal tea. I could eat as often and as much as I wanted as long as I strictly followed the food lists.

Curious about how to turn those restrictions into real meals, I studied the sample diet plan. Breakfast generally consisted of a meat such as bacon or sausage with spinach or avocado, a smoothie, or leftovers from dinner the night before. Fruit and vegetables were suggested as a snack three times a day, with a lunch of salad or lettuce wrap. Dinner was basically fish, stir fry, stew, or soup. There was even a chocolate coconut treat for dessert.

I was ready to get started!

Well, actually, I had to shop first. Using the recipes and the food guide, I prepared a grocery list unlike any I had ever used before.

About half of the items were produce!

The normal sole entry "bananas" on my weekly list was replaced with blueberries, strawberries, raspberries, apples, pears, peaches, cherries, plums, spinach, kale, artichoke, butternut squash, zucchini, beets, cabbage, celery, bok choy, romaine lettuce, sweet potatoes (aha, tuberous roots were okay), broccoli, cauliflower, avocado, shallots, asparagus, parsnips, cucumbers, radishes, regular-size carrots, and baby carrots.

Meats included turkey sausage, bacon, sliced turkey and roast beef, ground beef, chicken, tuna, salmon, mahimahi, and tilapia.

To complete the list, I jotted down unsweetened coconut milk, kombucha tea, kimchi, fermented pickles and sauerkraut, olive oil, oregano, basil, tarragon, thyme, coconut flakes, raw organic cocoa powder, coconut oil, stevia, and herbal tea. I noted the specific requirements for certain items such as uncured bacon, caffeine-free tea, and wild-caught fish.

I found a very large grocery store nearby that combined the organic market and conventional grocery store styles. It carried a huge variety of organic produce and contained a large section of organic, gluten-free, and non-GMO items, but also sold all the products I was used to seeing in my regular large-chain store. This was great for me since I didn't feel like either the organic market or the large chain store was a perfect fit.

Shopping took forever! Not only because I wasn't familiar with the layout of the enormous store, but also because I had never shopped for most of the items on my list. I didn't even know what some of them were! No doubt I spent more time in the produce section on that one day than I had spent in all previous shopping trips combined.

Eventually I found everything I needed once I figured out that shallots were little garlic-shaped onions, bok choy was cabbage, and parsnips were white carrots. I researched on my phone the difference between "natural" and "organic," the meaning and benefit of uncured pork, and followed a debate about whether grains fed to chickens would affect a celiac who ate the meat. Gluten protein in chicken meat appeared to be a controversial subject, but evidence leaned toward no significant effect on celiacs.

I didn't want to ignore the doctor's advice to avoid grain-fed chicken, but since I didn't find any grass-fed chicken in the store and had not yet found a farmer who grass-fed chickens, I really had no options. A number of the recipes on my new meal plan included chicken, so I wouldn't be able to follow the plan without it. I reasoned that maybe it wasn't critical since the plan was very specific about a number of requirements for other ingredients but made no reference to diet for the chicken meat. I selected an organic, hormone and antibiotic-free whole chicken and three large packages of chicken breasts, and hoped their feed wouldn't matter.

At home I unpacked the groceries and washed the produce. The vegetables alone covered the entire island in my kitchen! I had lots of cooking to do.

I started right away, determined to begin the new diet as soon as possible. I made a chicken stir fry with cabbage and zucchini, chicken soup with carrots and celery, and a tuna casserole with broccoli and cauliflower. I baked chicken breasts for lettuce wraps, fried ground beef with shallots to put on lettuce beds, baked sweet potatoes and butternut squash, and made a chocolate dessert with coconut flakes, coconut oil, and cocoa powder.

I was exhausted! But very, very happy. I had plenty of healthy food prepared and a meal plan for an entire week.

My first couple of days on the diet looked like this:

Day 1

Breakfast

- Two strips of bacon, some strawberries, an apple, a small cup of coffee (I knew I would have to stop drinking coffee during detox, but wasn't ready to give it up yet)

Snack

- Two turkey sausages, some baby carrots

Lunch

- Chicken stir fry

Snack

- Two apples, some fermented pickles, a cup of coffee

Dinner

- Romaine lettuce salad with salmon and shallots
- Smoothie with coconut milk, blueberries, strawberries, and raspberries
- Chocolate dessert
- Half a cup of coffee

Day 2

Breakfast

- Bacon with spinach, shallots, and avocado. A strawberry smoothie, a cup of mint tea

Snack

- Sauerkraut, sweet potato, a peach, a cup of coffee

Lunch

- Ground beef with shallots on lettuce, an apple, kombucha tea

Afternoon snack

- Lettuce wrap with turkey slices and avocado, some cherries, a cup of coffee

Dinner

- Tilapia with zucchini and shallots, ginger tea, chocolate dessert

I continued taking my regular daily medications: a thyroid drug, a pill for seasonal allergies, prescription anti-inflammatories, a stomach acid reducer to protect my intestinal lining from damage caused by the anti-inflammatory, plus pain medications. I had been taking ADD medications as needed, but tried not to take them at all to allow my adrenal glands to recover. I was working hard to replace my coffee habit with herbal tea for the same reason. I knew I would need to stop everything except the thyroid medication during detox.

For the next few days I continued with the diet plan. The food was absolutely delicious and very satisfying. With a few adjustments (such as removing radishes, yuck!), I thought I could live on the diet forever. I was surprised by how much I enjoyed eating butternut squash and sweet potatoes with a little cinnamon, and how I looked forward to a handful of pickle slices as a snack.

Spinach fried with bacon and shallots quickly became my breakfast favorite, and I actually craved a big salad of mixed greens, roast beef, avocado, and chopped apple. The combination of flavors was amazing. Pears baked with cinnamon and a little coconut oil was a fantastic dessert, as was the chocolate coconut treat.

The food was very different from anything I had eaten before, and every meal required much more effort than I was used to. It felt strange not to reach into a bag of chips for a snack or spread peanut butter on a slice of bread for lunch. But I truly appreciated knowing everything I put in my mouth was good for me and helping to improve my health.

I felt the physical effects of the drastic change in my diet, though. I was grumpy and tired off and on, and I craved sugar and carbs. I experienced headaches and muscle aches by the end of each day. While not exactly desirable, I didn't find these symptoms too disturbing since they were expected and would be temporary. Compared to a lifelong inability to explain or control my health issues, these discomforts were almost welcome since they signified a move in the direction I desperately wanted and sought for so long. I was no longer attempting to quiet my symptoms, I was truly healing my body.

After about a week on my new diet the detox kit arrived. It had so many supplements to keep track of, I was really glad I already had the diet part figured out! I wanted to start right away.

To begin preparing, I reread the detox section of the doctor's earlier email.

- Measure my blood pressure, heart rate, and weight every day so we have data to follow my progress. Journal every day. Detox can be difficult, and it can be helpful to capture experiences and emotions.
- Detox can cause strong reactions. I should go to the emergency room if urgently ill
- Eat every three to four hours; no food after 7:00 p.m.
- No more than fifty grams of carbs per day

I raided the family school supply stash and found a composition notebook, then stapled the doctor's instructions and the supplement guide for the detox program to the first few pages. I listed the supplements she recommended for pain and inflammation along with their doses on a big stickie note and added it to the supplement guide. Leaving the remaining front pages of the notebook empty for daily entries, I added to the back the lists of foods to eat and foods to avoid, recipes, and the sample diet plan.

I was ready.

The first couple of days were great! I had lots of energy and no pain, even without caffeine and my normal medications. But by the third day I was suffering from extreme back pain and an ache between my shoulder blades that hurt all day and kept me awake at night.

After a few days with no relief, I was exhausted and miserable. I quickly lost my optimistic perspective that welcomed slight discomforts as part of a bigger plan, and became desperate for a break. I experimented with a small amount of anti-inflammatory to see if it would help. It made a huge difference. I contacted my doctor to tell her my pain was nine out of ten all day and night without medication, and two out of ten with it.

She emphasized the importance of getting enough quality sleep, and said to take the smallest amount possible for a couple of days at bedtime so I could rest and my body could heal. She reminded me that anti-inflammatories damage intestinal lining, so I could not heal my gut if I continued to take them.

She thought my pain was likely the result of detox and was confident it would resolve in time. To get me through the worst symptoms, she increased the amount of fish oil I was taking and instructed me to get digestive enzymes, systemic enzymes, more herbal extracts for inflammation, and additional natural remedies for pain. Tea made with ginger and turmeric might bring some relief, and I should drink plenty of water.

With the new additions, my daily medication/supplement schedule looked like this:

6:00 a.m.: Thyroid medication on an empty stomach

7:00 a.m.: Enzymes for pain and inflammation on an empty stomach

8:00 a.m.: Fish oil, a natural painkiller, and a natural anti-inflammatory plus three plan supplement powders each dissolved in a full glass of water with breakfast

10:00 a.m.: Enzymes for pain and inflammation on an empty stomach

Noon: Fish oil, a natural painkiller, and a natural anti-inflammatory with lunch

2:00 p.m.: Enzymes for pain and inflammation on an empty stomach

5:00 p.m.: Fish oil, a natural pain killer, and two natural anti-inflammatories plus three plan supplement powders each dissolved in a full glass of water with dinner

Since beginning a gluten-free diet, I sometimes dreamed about eating something I shouldn't eat, usually pizza or a dessert. The dreams became much more frequent and unpleasant during detox. They didn't focus on the taste or satisfaction of eating delicious foods, but all centered on the terrible realization that I had consumed something that would damage my body and ruin my efforts to heal. They were so vivid that it took hours after waking for me to calm down and convince myself that I hadn't caused any harm. The kids told me they had similar dreams. Clearly the transition caused anxiety for all of us.

During the second phase of the detox program, I was feeling a little better. I had some cramping in my back muscles, a little joint pain, and was tired off and on, but overall felt pretty good. I was sleeping great, which made a huge difference in my energy and attitude. My daily supplements with breakfast and dinner increased to four powders dissolved in water and included two new supplements plus a packet of capsules.

After feeling pretty good for a number of days, I woke up one morning with severe muscle pain and was so exhausted I could hardly walk. I forced myself into the shower thinking that the water would wake me up and soothe my muscles, but turned the faucet off within a few seconds because I didn't have the energy to stand. I dried off and went back to bed.

For three days I couldn't go to work or do anything around the house. Desperate, and not really knowing what else to do, I increased the dose of my thyroid medication without my doctor's knowledge or guidance. I was convinced my extreme exhaustion was related to my thyroid, and taking more of a medication that was readily available was an easy solution. Consulting with the doctor seemed to require a herculean effort that I could not muster.

It made sense at the time.

During the last phase of the detox program, my pain and energy had improved, and I was back to work and almost normal function around the house. I still had cramps in my lower back, and was ill-tempered after weeks of feeling tired and uncomfortable.

The doctor didn't seem bothered by my grumpy one-word responses and minimal note-taking during a visit to review progress and discuss life after detox. She was encouraging and supportive, telling me I was doing a great job with the program and showing positive results.

While I was reluctant to initiate a conversation about thyroid medication, I had to confess to increasing my dose since I was running low and needed a refill. The doctor expressed that she was "very surprised" by my action and warned that taking more thyroid medication than I needed could damage my heart.

She gently explained that healing is a process that takes some time, and it is difficult sometimes to wait.

I grunted under my breath. "Difficult"?

The pain alone was incapacitating, but the weakness I experienced prevented even the most basic activity. Did she know that?

In fairness, I didn't tell her or ask for her advice. I was in no mood to admit fault. I guess I did not yet trust that a medical professional understood what I needed and could help me. Or maybe I had just been impatient to feel better.

As I silently fumed over my challenging experience, she explained that the leg cramps I recently developed were likely due to an imbalance caused by the excessive thyroid medication. She suggested some additional supplements to address the issue.

When I dropped my dose of thyroid medication back to the prescribed amount, I felt much less irritable and my typical optimistic perspective returned.

Humbled and more than a little shaken by my disregard for consequences, I vowed to no longer practice medicine and would at least consult the doctor before deciding she wouldn't help me.

I would try to trust her.

Chapter Twenty

SLOW PROGRESS

Suddenly detox was over.

No more powders or pill packets to manage, no need to capture thoughts and actions in my red notebook. I finished the six-week program thirteen pounds lighter than when I started, and my blood pressure dropped from about 130/70 prior to the program to consistently about 80/60 after.

The doctor provided instructions about what foods to avoid permanently and how to slowly introduce some foods back to my diet. She recommended paleo cookbooks to expand my meal options and suggested eating organ meat such as heart and liver as well as preparing broth from bones. She listed supplements I should take as maintenance going forward, and provided tips for eating while traveling. We would meet a couple of times each year to see how I was doing.

After years of searching for answers, I was a bit stunned to realize that I had the recipe for my health and was well on my way toward achieving it. I had not only eliminated damaging food and medications, I was also nourishing my body with the right supplements and healthy meals. I was sleeping very well and hoped to add exercise back into my daily routine once my joint and muscle pain lessened. While I was disappointed that I didn't feel drastically better physically, I understood that my symptoms would continue to improve over time.

I didn't experiment much right away with adding new foods to my diet. Since Kenny and Chris discovered that they felt great eating what I was eating, I was cooking plenty of food I really enjoyed and knew wouldn't bother me. I didn't really feel a need to expand my options. It was summertime and we were planning a vacation as well as preparing Kenny for college in the fall, so I had more than enough activities to keep me busy without making an effort to try food I thought might irritate my fragile state.

We tried to maintain our diet while on vacation, but found it very difficult to prepare meals away from home and to manage ingredients while eating out. We stocked our mini refrigerator with food from an organic market and ordered plain meat and vegetables at restaurants, but had only limited control over cross-contamination and hidden additives. At the end of the trip I ate something that caused a strong reaction, and returned home with terrible back cramps, joint pain, difficulty focusing, and exceptional fatigue. With only one day to recover before Kenny's college orientation, I was in a poor state to start this milestone event.

I'd attended the same orientation with Gretchen two years earlier, and was thrilled to share a similar experience with Kenny. The informational sessions and impressive speakers were highly motivating, and I expected that they would infuse Kenny with pride and excitement about the next four years of life at a large university.

Kenny, possibly also affected by food on our trip, uncharacteristically slept for the early-morning two-hour drive to the school as I tried my best to rally for a full day of presentations and socialization. Kenny would be staying overnight in a dormitory as part of his student orientation, while I would leave in the evening and return the next day to attend the remaining parent activities and to pick Kenny up. Since Chris was home alone and the distance was manageable, I declined the option to remain in the area for the night.

After a few hours of shuffling between buildings for tours and sitting through lectures about move-in day and the risks and statistics of underage drinking, my back clamped in a painful spasm and I was falling asleep on my feet. I felt incapable of making conversation or absorbing information and was desperate to find somewhere to rest. I responded to Kenny's text messages about taking a German placement exam and the opportunity for a night-time hike, then left my group of parents.

I walked across campus checking out shady spots under trees and wondering about the possibility of finding a dorm room or lecture hall that was unlocked and empty where I could lie down. I found myself at my car in a parking garage on the far edge of the college's grounds. I knew I couldn't drive. Instead I climbed into the backseat, shoving grocery bags and jumper cables into the fold of the seats to create a flat surface where I could stretch out on my back without my spine sagging painfully. I was so uncomfortable I didn't think I would be able to take the short nap I desperately wanted.

I held the orientation schedule above my head and reviewed it again and again, unable to decide what to do next. Overwhelmed with frustration and concerned that I would disappoint Kenny by not participating, I dropped the schedule to the floor and looked out the back window. Tears slid down my cheeks as I considered whether I should return to the sessions or just drive home once the pain weakened and I regained the energy to move.

Groaning with pain, I sat up suddenly and looked at my watch. I'd slept for almost five hours. Realizing that an urgent need to urinate had woken me up, I quickly exited the car. Shoeless and with a single focus on the pain of my extremely full bladder, I scanned my surroundings in a panic. I could see nothing nearby that would serve my need. No gas stations, restaurants, or even construction sites with a portable restroom. As I eyed a very small cluster of trees and imagined being spotted with my shorts down by a group of touring parents, my bladder released with an unstoppable flow.

I looked around frantically. The fact that I didn't spot any people or cameras provided only minimal comfort. I hoped my open car door would provide some protection if someone appeared, but knew there would be no hiding the truth from anyone within sight. Or sound.

It was not one of my better moments.

I spread grocery bags on the driver's seat and drove home. I was humiliated and soaked with pee. By the time I stopped for gas an hour later, I no longer cared if anyone noticed my wet clothes or smelled the urine. I didn't want to think about it. I just wanted to go home, take a shower, and go to bed.

As I drove I reflected on the conversation with my doctor when she told me it could take a year to feel better and that waiting was difficult. It was! It was difficult waiting for my thyroid medication to stabilize, waiting for my leaky gut to heal, waiting for the pain to go away. It would be so easy to just take something! Pain pills, caffeine, ADD medication, anti-inflammatories. Any of these would have made me feel better immediately. They were proven remedies and expected treatments. I didn't even know if leaky gut was real. Could I wait a year to find out? Everyone I talked to about what I was doing thought I was insane. Was I? Did I need to put myself through this?

Once I was clean and rested, I admitted to myself that I was not ready to abandon the course I had chosen and destroy all my hard work. I knew there would be short-term sacrifices for a long-term solution, and I recommitted to making them. I would give my body a fair chance to heal. My plan of action made sense. I would not give it up so soon.

A few weeks later, I was still suffering from terrible pain and fatigue when I visited Gretchen for her birthday. She lived in an apartment off campus and was preparing for the upcoming semester.

I felt distracted, but, as always, uplifted by spending time with Gret. I was able to make our traditional run to IHOP, where she had a gluten-free country omelet and I had a glass of water. It would be a while before I was going to take any risks with food. I watched her eat as we discussed dates and crushes, whether she should try for captain of the ultimate Frisbee team, and the opportunity for a semester abroad.

On the trip home, my sense of desperation became overwhelming as I struggled to find a bearable position. My joints were screaming and my neck and back were twisted with spasms that were not at all lessened by anything I did. I tried every possible adjustment of the seat and arrangement of my body with and without cushions under and behind me, but nothing helped. I felt like I had no control, no ability to make myself feel better. I wanted to pull over and sleep, but there was a list of things waiting for me to do at home and I didn't really think stopping would help anyway.

As I fidgeted and fumed, I heard on the radio that actor/comedian Robin Williams had committed suicide. I was shocked. It was reported that he suffered from depression and substance abuse. Apparently just before his death he had reentered rehab for "maintenance." He wasn't taking drugs at the time. I had absolutely no idea what his life was like, but as the radio described celebrity reactions to his death, I thought about what he might have been experiencing.

Maybe he didn't feel right, which was affecting his quality of life. There was something he could "take" to feel better, but those things were forbidden. I'd heard that people commit suicide when they believe there is no other option. That it's the result of having no hope.

For me, I might have felt ashamed or embarrassed about taking medications because I would feel like I had given up and because I might have been delaying my healing. But in truth I could have taken what I needed to feel better and nobody would have cared.

What I needed was legal, cheap, and widely accepted. Encouraged, in fact. Plus, I was optimistic that my struggle was temporary. I wondered what I would do if things were different.

What if I had no hope of ever relieving my pain, or what if the only help was prohibited or would negatively affect the people I love? Could I live in pain with no hope? Or would I do what I had to do to get through the day, knowing that I was hurting myself and others?

What a horribly devastating battle! I was very still and quiet the rest of the way home as I mourned an actor I didn't know and imagined the lives of people facing every day without hope.

Chapter Twenty-One

PLAYING WITH FOOD

During the summer, the kids and I began to experiment with expanding our food options. We didn't want to reintroduce any known sensitivities, but we were interested in finding a little more variety. For a peanut butter sandwich and potato chips type of gal whose previous idea of cooking was to stir chopped hot dogs into a can of beans or to melt American cheese on top of a dish of macaroni, ground beef, and pasta sauce, I was still getting used to the idea that I could keep the family alive on fresh produce and meats.

As we investigated new recipes and different types of diets, I realized how limited my view had been and what an amazing variety of healthy foods were available to us.

For our first phase of experimentation we played it safe, selecting dinner recipes that avoided inflammatory foods but included elements that were new to us. I considered this our fancy phase, since the dishes seemed better suited for a special occasion than an everyday meal. While I had grown accustomed to the new foods introduced through detox since they remained a major part of our diet, I still felt that a meal was extravagant if it included a meat other than beef or chicken, a vegetable other than potatoes or green beans, or was seasoned with something other than salt and pepper.

During our fancy phase we made pork tenderloin marinated in olive oil and coconut nectar, rosemary-roasted lamb, and ginger-baked salmon. For sides we tried mint zucchini, sweet potatoes mashed with coconut oil and topped with shredded coconut, fried cauliflower with turmeric and ginger, and a colorful dish of baked parsnips, carrots, beets, and rutabaga. We boiled artichoke then grilled it with olive oil, and baked dates wrapped in bacon. Some recipes we made only once; others, many times. One that became a fast favorite and a regular dish in our house was Brussels sprouts with crispy bacon and a little apple cider vinegar.

Our second round of experimentation was the baking phase. We missed having bread, and the commercial products available contained many ingredients we didn't want to eat. Using grain-free flours such as almond, coconut, tapioca, plantain, cassava, and sweet potato, we conducted dozens of trials resulting in a huge variety of products, but none that came close to resembling what we thought of as bread. The bread we made was not white, not light, and not tall. In fact, what we made were usually dark, heavy, flat batches of something that looked more like brownies than bread. When we did create a loaf-like product, the slices were dry and about the size of a small cracker.

Once we finally let go of our concept of bread as sandwich slices or something we could put in the toaster, we landed on a recipe for a type of flatbread that we baked in a thick layer on a cookie sheet. The "bread" was made of almond flour, arrowroot, coconut milk, flaxseed, applesauce, agave, and apple cider vinegar, and was heavy, nutty, sweet, moist, and delicious. We eventually scaled the recipe to make huge batches, cut it into two-inch squares, and devoured it with abandon. It didn't make a good sandwich because it was too thick and crumbly, but it was delicious hot, cold, by itself, or topped with honey. It became a routine preparation in our kitchen, which was constantly covered in a fine layer of arrowroot powder.

Other than feeling extremely uncomfortable after gorging ourselves on the almond bread, we had no adverse reaction to our baking. With a renewed sense of confidence and adventure, our efforts expanded to include other sweet items. It was fun to play with new recipes when the food wasn't required for our survival! These were treats, completely unnecessary and indulgent.

We found during our quest for bread that paleo recipes were a good fit for us, and we were amazed by the number and variety of options. Some came with entertaining stories about entire families following this hunter/gatherer diet without their knowledge, since Mom prepared all the food and thought the approach was good for them but didn't think they would support the limitations and odd substitutions if they knew.

We made wonderful cookies, cakes, and icing from different combinations of coconut flour, coconut oil, vanilla, and honey. With varying success we also tried gingerbread cookies made from almond flour, brownies of cassava flour and cocoa powder, coconut balls with agave and vanilla, and fig coconut bites with cinnamon. We even made ice cream using coconut milk and avocado! The sweets all tasted good, though the appearance did not always meet our expectations. No doubt the discrepancy was due to a lack of attention to detail by the enthusiastic bakers rather than flawed instructions. A couple of recipes with consistently good outcomes in flavor and form that became house favorites were fresh carrot apple cinnamon muffins, and pumpkin muffins with dairy-free chocolate chips.

When Gretchen and Kenny returned to college full time at the end of the summer, I was happy to dial back the pursuit of new foods and settle in to routine food preparation for Chris and myself. We were content with the variety we had established, and I was hoping we could spend a little more time outside the house. Kenny, though, excited to have a kitchen to himself and interested in extending the exploration, continued to look for alternatives.

Deviating from our earlier style of experimentation bursts, we entered a new, extended phase where Kenny would discover something new and convince the rest of us to try it.

Kenny introduced us to tiger nuts, a little tuber that originated as an important crop in ancient Egypt, expanded internationally mostly as a weed, and became popular with paleo dieters because of its high fiber and calcium content. The "nuts" looked to me like wrinkled peanuts but were surprisingly sweet and chewy. *Very* chewy. I tried soaking them in water to plump them up and enjoyed them as a snack when they were hydrated, but found they made my stomach crampy and never really incorporated them into my diet.

Kenny also discovered miso, jars of very flavorful fermented azuki beans and chickpeas we ate with a spoon every few days rather than adding it to a dish or using it to make soup, as I think it was intended. I thought of miso more as healthy bacteria rather than a snack or part of a meal, and kept a few jars of the thick, chunky paste in the house for use as a probiotic supplement.

Kenny had previously been guided to new and different foods by internet research, but one day he called me out of the blue with a discovery.

"Mom, you won't believe it! There are SO many foods we can eat!"

I was confused. Kenny, always considerate, never called without first sending a text to see if I was available. And we never talked in the middle of the afternoon when I was at work.

"I've been eating so little for so long and now there's so much more!" he said. "The vegetables here are amazing!"

I thought I heard traffic in the background. "Where are you?"

"I'm in the parking lot at the international market! I'm sending you photos!" He had a little spring in his voice, like he was bouncing on his feet.

I closed my office door and put Kenny on speaker. The photos came through one after another, *ping, ping, ping,* each one a different bag in Kenny's trunk with leafy vegetables poking out.

"Can you see everything?" he asked. "We can eat it all! You've got to get some of this!"

Kenny was a serious student with sights on graduate school, so he limited his diet to what he knew was safe. He didn't want to eat anything that would affect his schoolwork or cause him to miss class.

I enlarged the photos to see if I could recognize the vegetables.

"I've been working off such a short list of foods I can eat," he said, "and such a long list of ones I can't. Now the list of what I can eat is huge! It's fantastic!!"

I enjoyed hearing about Kenny's adventures with new foods. Finally giving in to his pleas, I began to visit international markets in our area. I curiously explored the entire store, but limited my purchases to produce, since I wasn't really sure about the ingredients in packaged products and didn't want to eat anything that would cause irritation to my still very sensitive back.

Maybe I spent too much time considering the items when I shopped, because I regularly received very welcome advice from other shoppers on how to select or prepare the food. In the vegetable area, for example, I learned that jicama and batata can be eaten raw and make great snacks, while taro is toxic when raw but delicious and nutritious when boiled and mashed.

Good to know!

After much baking, boiling, and mashing, Chris and I didn't really find any vegetables that we couldn't live without. Until we tried frying. We bought a little fry pot and made chips out of batata, parsnip, sweet potatoes, taro, beets, and jicama, which became a huge hit in our house. They were fantastic! Crunchy, salty, and sweet, they were unlike anything else we had in our diet.

The chips were a huge failure, however, in my efforts to simplify food production. The chip-making process was quite extensive and time-consuming. We washed and peeled the vegetables, sliced them with a mandoline slicer (eventually using slice-resistant gloves after a couple of nasty incidents involving my fingers), then put the slices in bowls of ice water to chill so they would be firm. We quickly dried small batches, fried them in olive oil, then spread them out on paper towels to dry again, sprinkled with salt. They really were delicious. Eventually we limited the vegetables to only batatas because they stayed crunchy for days after cooking and were relatively easy to prepare since we didn't have to peel them or soak them in ice water. Unwilling to give them up regardless of the effort they required, we added chips to our list of weekend large-batch productions, along with almond bread and stir fry.

I started making bone broth at home because of my doctor's ravings about its nutritional benefits and ability to reduce inflammation, improve skin, slow aging, and promote sound sleep, which were echoed by Kenny and numerous internet commenters. The winning attribute for me was the anti-inflammatory properties, which would not only help heal my leaky gut but also promised to reduce my joint pain. Unable to find commercial broths that met my need for a minimal number of ingredients, I convinced myself that this additional very involved process was worth the effort.

To make the broth I first boiled bones in a huge pot of water, skimming gray foam off the top as it appeared and dropping it into the trash. I then roasted the bones in a very hot oven, transferred them with the little crispy pieces that fell out during baking into a Crock-Pot, filled the Crock-Pot with water, and added apple cider vinegar to help free the nutrients from the bones. We experimented with adding vegetables and herbs in different combinations to the water at this stage, but found that thoroughly roasted bones created the best flavor without any additional ingredients.

After bringing the Crock-Pot water to a boil, I reduced it to a simmer for three days and it required no attention other than adding more water every few hours to keep the bones covered.

The Crock-Pot generated so much heat that in the summertime I had to move the simmering operation to the garage. After three days, I poured the savory broth through a strainer into a roasting pan with a couple of cubes of ice to cool the liquid quickly and reduce the risk of bacteria growth. I then ladled the cooled broth into plastic cups with lids and placed half in the freezer and half in the refrigerator.

When we first undertook the bone broth initiative I thought the most difficult part of the process would be finding the organic, grass-fed beef bones the doctor recommended. Finding them actually was the difficult part of the process, but not because stores didn't carry them. They were difficult to find because butcher shops and grocery stores sold out as soon as the bones arrived. I wondered who was buying them and if they were all used to make broth. What else could you do with them?

I was again struck by the sense that there was a large movement going on around me that I wanted to understand but didn't know how to find. Were there people close by with health experiences similar to mine, trying to discover what their bodies needed and how to provide it so they could function at their best?

Maybe that was just wishful thinking and the people buying the bones were making broth as a traditional part of their diet or simply trying out a new fad. But why would someone who is not supersensitive exert the effort to get bones from organic, grass-fed beef? Bone broth can be made from any kind of bones, and the typical consumer wouldn't likely need them to be organic or grass-fed, would they? Chicken, turkey, ham, or rib bones are commonly used for broth and readily available as leftovers.

During the several months I left work at lunchtime to intercept the delivery of fresh bones at a local butcher shop, I half expected to meet my soulmate in line. But I never met anyone else, and eventually discovered that I could usually find one or two bags of frozen bones at the organic market near my house if I went after work on the day of the delivery. I never met anyone shopping for those either.

The bone-buying people probably would have thought nothing of the matching practices Kenny and I adopted of cooking beef liver in a small, round convection oven on the kitchen counter. It cooked much more quickly and more evenly than the big oven, and the clear cover allowed us to keep a close eye on the batch's progress. Our friends who gawked at the soft, purple-red lobes sagging between the rack's thin wires and dripping juices onto the base clearly did not have a pot of bone broth brewing in their garage.

By this time I was pretty sure I had replaced all of the hygienic products in the house with gluten-free options and was generally happy with their effectiveness, though the natural deodorant I used contained some ingredient that every dog I was ever around wanted to taste. I first realized this during an office Christmas party when the host's 150-pound mastiff was obsessed with burying his nose in my armpit. My coworkers were thoroughly entertained by his persistence as I awkwardly tried to push him away all evening, leaving with slobber and snot all over my blouse.

The biggest product replacement win was finding the right toothpaste, which put an end to my chronic mouth sores. More than two years after discovering gluten, I had finally reached a point where I wasn't struggling to control the factors affecting my health.

But I wasn't as active or agile as I had hoped. I still had lingering pain, and figured my joints were damaged by decades of chronic inflammation.

I thought they would always bother me.

Chapter Twenty-Two

MY SOLUTION

My doctor was still troubled by my unresolved pain and constant low level of autoimmune activity, and continued to look for possible causes. I went through additional testing for food sensitivities, gut bacteria imbalance, and nutrient deficiencies. This resulted in small changes to my supplements and diet but did not resolve my issues.

Over time I began to realize that some of the foods I was consuming regularly were bothering me. Through a very long process of discovery and elimination, I eventually removed coconut, fermented foods, pumpkin, almond bread (I couldn't identify the specific problematic ingredient), and chocolate from my diet completely.

I also limited my frequency of eating some other foods, such as sweet potatoes and broccoli. While I experienced an obvious reduction in joint pain, the resolution was not complete. My vanity, however, led me to the final piece of the puzzle.

While I was at the dentist's office for a regular cleaning, the hygienist commented that my teeth were badly stained from drinking tea. All my life I had been complimented on the whiteness of my teeth, so I was disturbed by the effect of my recently acquired tea habit. I drank it several times every day for its health benefits, not because I was particularly attached to it.

I decided I would try not drinking tea at all and see what happened. The next day, after skipping three or four cups, I was shocked to find that my pain was completely resolved and I was full of energy. I had never felt better in my life! I was nimble and flexible, with no tightness or soreness. I could move without fear of causing a cramp, and could sit without a sickening ache in my lower back. I couldn't believe it! I had an almost irresistible desire to do cartwheels.

For the next few days I bounced around telling anyone who would listen how good I felt and how surprised I was that the solution was so simple. My new boss at work was supportive but weary as I pointed out every new discovery.

"Look!" I said as she attempted to start a staff meeting. "I can twist around in my chair. I'm sitting and twisting!"

Then I sat sideways in the bucket seat of her car on the way to an offsite meeting. "Look! I'm just sitting in this weird position without squirming or complaining. I can bend over and touch my toes!"

She truly was happy for me. She knew about my struggle and the importance of my new discovery.

"Just tell me where to turn," she said with a huge smile.

At the end of that week on Friday night, a calm settled over me that was different from anything I'd ever experienced. I sat by myself on our deck as the sun set and let the significance of my realization soak in. Since the first step in regaining my health was an accidental discovery, it seemed appropriate that the last step was also found by chance.

I marveled at my fortunate decision to follow my friend Prancer's diet years before, and shuddered at the memory of my condition at that time and at the realization of what my life would have been like had I not acted on the whim to try what she was eating.

Long after dark, Chris came out to see if I was okay and to ask if he should eat dinner without me. I gazed at the beautiful stars and felt that time was standing still. I wasn't hungry, I wasn't tired, I wasn't uncomfortable. I had actually ended my body's lifelong process of self- destruction. I felt that I had at last finished a race I had been running my entire life, but had no interest in a rowdy celebration.

I was at peace.

Late into the night, I just sat and quietly enjoyed the absence of struggle and fear. I felt whole. I chuckled as I thought about my earlier powerful impulse to perform cartwheels, a simple move I couldn't execute even as a child.

With a consistent baseline of no pain, clear focus, and an abundance of energy, I was able to test my specific reaction to different foods. I wanted to know if I could be less cautious about eating out, if I could replace some of my home-cooked meals with store-bought ones, and if I could add back any of the foods I had excluded from my diet. I had no plans to ever eat dairy or gluten, but wanted to go through the typical progressive process for reintroducing foods that I had postponed following the detox diet because of my ongoing symptoms.

I tried one new food at a time and carefully watched for a reaction for several days. I found that my most typical adverse reactions were incredible bloating with an impressive five- pound overnight weight gain, severe and frequent hot flashes, debilitating joint pain that lasted for three days or more, muscle weakness, exhaustion, an inability to focus, and irritability. Less frequent but clearly reproducible reactions included a racing pulse, insomnia, acne, muscle aches, noticeably limp hair, feeling very cold, sinus congestion, uncontrolled hunger, dozens of tiny clear blisters on my hands, wheezing, a feeling of detachment, stomach ache, and headache.

While not exactly fun, the ability to definitively pinpoint a food with a symptom was very satisfying.

Over the course of many months, I developed a good under-standing of my response to a number of foods. Consistent, clear, very negative results convinced me that I could absolutely not tolerate grains, yeast, vinegar, alcohol, coffee, tea, fermented foods or drinks, any type of added sugar (including agave and honey), eggs, soy, sesame oil, guar gum and xanthan gum (food additives), and several over-the-counter medications.

I could tolerate other foods in moderation, including toma-toes, beans, peppers, onions, avocados, apples, bananas, grapes, citrus fruit, carrots, pumpkin seeds, root vegetables, chicken, sar-dines, salmon, broccoli, sweet potatoes, white potatoes, peanuts, cashews, macadamia nuts, raisins, coconut, pumpkin, almonds, and chocolate.

I was able to eat unlimited amounts of beef and, surprisingly, white rice. White rice was possibly not an ideal staple food from a nutritional perspective, but I needed carbohydrates and was unable to find another good source. I thought maybe I was able to tolerate white rice because the husk, bran, and grain were removed, eliminating elements that would normally cause an immune reaction. White rice, ground beef, and green, leafy veg-etables (usually kale or collard greens) fried in olive oil became my go-to meal that I could eat every day without issue. I rotated through the other foods I could tolerate in limited amounts to avoid a negative reaction but still have some diversity in my diet.

I considered that I might be the most sensitive person in the world, but truly appreciated being aware of the effect of food on my body. For almost fifty years I never thought about anything I popped in my mouth and just ate whatever food was available and appealing. I had definitely learned to think about what I ate to avoid harm, but the process of discovering my sensitivities also taught me to consider what my body needed to function.

During a routine visit with my doctor, I proudly described the findings of my experimentation and the successful elimination of problematic foods. She asked a number of questions, identified possible causes for some of the sensitivities, provided resources for additional information, and discussed testing for me to consider. She was very complimentary of my efforts and praised my success in eliminating inflammation and pain.

Just as I was about to pat myself on the back for being the smartest person in the world, however, she began to explain the results of our recent nutrient testing.

She circled little arrows on a diagram that indicated where nutrients enter critical metabolic processes. She explained in detail how insufficient amounts of those nutrients affect the body's ability to generate energy and remove toxins.

I realized that I never before considered how my body actually worked and what it might need from me to function effectively. Her illustration made the mysterious internal workings of my body real, and showed very clearly that each step was dependent on the availability of some essential element to move forward.

How did I get so far in life without ever thinking about what was going on inside me and what I needed to do to make sure it went well? I'd studied these cycles in school and could probably even answer some basic questions about requirements and results. How had I not made a connection between what I learned and what my body needed to operate?

I'd just assumed that I was fine doing what everybody else around me was doing with their food and lifestyle, and that a doctor would fix me if I was sick. More recently I'd learned that I could do things to avoid problems for myself, but even then I never felt accountable for making sure things went right.

The realization I experienced as her scientific textbook image transformed into a living part of me changed my entire perspective and forced me to think about my role differently. I wanted to know what I could do to truly take care of myself and provide what my body needed to be as healthy as possible.

My broadened awareness allowed me to finally recognize the more direct nudges from my doctor for what they were, and I began to take ownership for all aspects of my health. Not only nutrition, but also sleep, exercise, and reducing stress in my life. I evaluated my job, my relationships, and how I spent my time, then made a number of significant positive changes.

I found that my wants were more habits than true desires. I was amazed at how happy and content I felt when I ate foods that were right for me, exercised regularly, slept for eight hours every night, worked a job I enjoyed, and spent time with people who supported me.

Historically I had struggled with an incredibly strong desire for an immediate solution to any small complaint. Even after I changed my diet and felt much better, I still wanted to pop a pill the instant I had a hint of a headache, drink alcohol when I was grumpy or wanted to be more social, eat junk food when I was bored, or drink caffeine when I wanted more energy.

Once I settled into my new lifestyle, my compulsion for quick fixes went away. I still sometimes considered an easy remedy for some minor discomfort, but my old habits no longer dominated my thoughts. I was able to easily ignore the issue and employ a better solution.

I'll admit that I continued to search for a source of caffeine, since I still lived in a world where I couldn't always get enough sleep and sometimes needed to function when I was tired. I occasionally struggled to stay awake during an unusually early morning meeting at work, or when driving home after a long day out with the kids. Ironically, almost every substance with caffeine and even pure caffeine capsules made me foggy and groggy. I did eventually find a brand of caffeine water that was effective in small amounts, and kept a few bottles available at work and home for use when I needed them.

Without physical distractions and with the return of my natural abundance of energy, I felt like my true self for the first time in many, many years.

Gretchen and Kenny were away at school most of the time, but Chris became my willing partner-in-crime for projects around the house and fun activities in the area. We rebuilt our dilapidated farm-style fence with pickets that more effectively prevented the escape of our little dog Bentley. I genuinely marveled at my ease of movement with every bend and squat to place each of the five hundred boards around the perimeter of the yard. We landscaped the lawn, cleaned out closets and the garage, replaced old toilets, and repainted most of the house. When the weather was nice, we forgot our long list of home improvement projects and hiked trails along the Potomac River or boarded the Metro to tour museums and monuments in the nation's capital.

Chris and I joined a gym and worked out five or six days a week, taking cardio classes or hopping on a stair machine or stationary bike when the classes were too full. When Gret and Kenny were home we all exercised together, bumping into each other in the living room as we followed whatever intense interval training video they were using at the time. Eventually I could almost keep up with the endless planks, push-ups, mountain climbers, punches, kicks, burpees, and lunges with just a few modifications to accommodate my damaged joints. I normally didn't feel pain during or after a workout, but I could definitely irritate my back, knees, and hips with too many twists or high jumps.

For longer school breaks we all piled in the car to go to the beach or to spend a few days boating and fishing with a friend who lived on a nearby lake. Whether they were lazily lounging around the house in the morning or passionately debating a board game rule at night, I cherished every second of my time with the kids. I remembered very clearly the days in the not so distant past when I was so overwhelmed with pain and exhaustion that I was angered by their need for my attention. The memory of those times sickened me, and I was so incredibly thankful for the events and people that helped me to find another way.

I could still conjure up memories of a weak, confused, terribly miserable, and self-absorbed person trying desperately to address a multitude of issues and get through the day, but it was difficult to believe that person was me. I remembered the fear and frustration of knowing that so many symptoms must have indicated a serious underlying issue but not being able to identify what it was.

All of those symptoms were gone. My hands and feet were warm and soft, with no cracking or peeling. There were no dry patches on my sides, bumps on my skin, or sores in my mouth. I didn't catch whatever cold or flu was going around, and my twice-a-year sinus infections were history. I had no stabbing pain in my abdomen when I rolled out of bed, no urgent need to pee every hour, and no blood in my urine during routine exams. None of my joints hurt and I no longer had any signs of carpal tunnel syndrome. I couldn't nap during the day if I tried, but slept soundly through the night regardless of my position. I felt strong and capable, patient and understanding. I was focused and engaged in my work.

I felt like a different person. But this person was me! The despondent person from my memory with pills in her pockets and booze by her bed was someone else.

I hadn't been sick in more than three years, but I still met with traditional medicine physicians for preventive exams and to address degenerated joints. My joints were no longer inflamed, but surgical intervention was sometimes needed to repair damage and remove debris. I had become so accustomed to the open, respectful, logical, and informative discussions with my functional medicine doctor that the prescribed and crisp nature of traditional physicians was often shocking in comparison.

One example of these experiences came when I was due for a routine colonoscopy. A new doctor in the practice I'd been to before entered the exam room, clipboard in hand, and sat at a small table next to me. She was a stern-looking woman, with deep furrows between her eyebrows and straight, dark hair pulled into a very tight knot at the back of her head.

"So what brings you here today?" she asked pleasantly.

I was happy for a simple goal that was not controversial. "Hi. I had a colonoscopy here a few years ago and I am due for another one."

She flipped through her papers. "Any changes to your medical history since you were here last?"

Uh-oh. I really just wanted to schedule a colonoscopy, not trigger a lecture on grains in my diet. But I thought a digestive disorder was probably relevant.

I studied her. "I might be a celiac."

She looked up from her clipboard. "What makes you think you are a celiac?"

I hesitated, wondering what to say to get through the questions as easily as possible. "Well, I had a lot of medical issues that went away when I stopped eating gluten."

"I see," she said. "Did you have an endoscopy?"

"No," I said, hoping to avoid controversy, "it's not a confirmed diagnosis."

She nodded. "Well then, we should get an endoscopy too. Celiacs have a much higher incidence of stomach cancer, so I'd like to take a look and make sure everything is okay."

Oh, whew! She didn't challenge my story, and I would get an actual report on the condition of my villi!

"That's great!" I said with new optimism, feeling that we were on the same team. "I've been working hard to heal my gut and would love to know how it looks and if it still shows signs of damage."

She wrote something on her clipboard, then said, "We *will* see damage if you are a celiac. Celiacs never successfully remove gluten from their diet."

Her comment surprised me. I squinted, trying to decide if I was offended as she left the room.

I had the procedures and anxiously waited for the results. A few weeks later I received a card in the mail that said, "Results normal. Next colonoscopy three years."

I called the office to ask about the results of the endoscopy. The receptionist put me on hold for a few minutes, then said, "The nurse says there are no notes from the doctor, so I guess you are fine."

"Is there any kind of report I can get from the procedure?" I asked, still hoping for some information.

She put me on hold again while she checked with the nurse. "There is a pathology report. Do you want me to mail a copy to you?"

"Yes, please," I said as I tried to suppress my disappointment with the time it would take to receive it.

About a week later, I received the report, containing a page and a half of descriptions and diagnoses. I looked up a number of the terms but couldn't comprehend their significance. I saw "reactive gastropathy" and "regenerative change" as well as a number of other findings I wanted to understand better.

I scheduled a follow-up appointment with the GI doctor to review the results.

I sat in the same small room, report and notepad in hand, waiting for the doctor to join me.

She walked in looking confused and a little frustrated. She flipped through her papers and said, "Why are you here? Your results are fine. I didn't request a follow-up."

"I was hoping you could explain the pathology report to me. I would love to know what you found during the endoscopy."

She laughed. "You came here because you want me to explain a report to you? I can't believe it. You are fine." She shook her papers in the air. "You had a normal reaction to the prep procedure. This is a waste of my time."

She turned and walked out.

I just sat there, looking at the report in my hands. I was frustrated that I took time off work and spent money for an appointment that was not only useless to me but also insulting, and disappointed that I could not form a partnership I truly wanted with my doctor.

After a number of similar interactions with traditional physicians, I simply quit trying to have two-way conversations. I learned to explain the reason for my visit as briefly as possible, and ignore the attitude of the person providing my care. I had confidence in what I'd learned about myself and my health, so I was no longer unnerved by their lack of support. But I always regretted that I couldn't have an open and honest conversation about what I needed to be healthy with a professional who was caring for me.

Chapter Twenty-Three

TODAY

My alarm woke me up at 6:00 a.m. and I sprang out of bed, ready to start a busy day. I let the dogs out into the yard and quickly showered, then ate a bowl of chicken and rice standing at the kitchen island while I scooped stir fry into a container for lunch. As I drove to work I reviewed a mental checklist to make sure I was prepared for the first few hours of activities.

Twenty new problem solvers were graduating from their three-week training class, and as lead for the program I needed to make sure everything was ready. Copies of the final exam were in a folder at my desk, and the room was set up with additional chairs for the leadership team who would join us for project presentations. Certificates were signed and meals were ordered for the lunch celebration. I just need to make sure extra tables were set up in the back of the room for the food.

After lunch I would present my own project to the leadership team. I'd been working for three months to shorten the time needed to deliver results to a client once laboratory testing was complete, which would improve client satisfaction, make our company more competitive, and increase our capacity for more work. We achieved a 70 percent decrease in reporting time, and I looked forward to discussing the approach and results with leaders. Slides were prepared, and I'd practiced my presentation as well as my response to a number of possible questions. I was ready.

The day flew by without a hitch. By late afternoon I was at my desk and working my way through email. I sent a message to my boss, who was traveling, to let her know that everyone passed the exam and all the projects were well received. In a few weeks we would start another wave of trainees, who would need new projects. I was already thinking about how we could build on the ones that were wrapping up.

One of the leaders who attended my presentation called and said he wanted me to leverage my report generation project to other service lines throughout the company. As I considered the logistics and planned my next steps, I realized it was 4:00 p.m. and time to leave so I could get Chris to karate class by 5:00 p.m.

I dropped him off at the door with just enough time to take off his shoes and line up before class began. I ran to the pet store for dog food, picked Chris up, then enjoyed an evening of tennis and dinner with the kids.

It was getting late by the time I packed lunches for the next day and let the dogs into the yard, but I still followed them out and sat on the deck to enjoy a few more minutes of the spring air. I slid down in the chair and rested my head on the cool metal back. I loved how normal my life had become. Three years ago I didn't think I would even be alive today. Now I packed my day with as much activity as I wanted, without a thought about whether I would be able to do whatever I had planned. I had zero complaints, no cause for hesitation at work or at home.

When I came back into the house with the dogs I paused for a minute to watch the kids piled on the living room couch, laughing at each other and the television. I kissed them good night, which they tolerated, then headed upstairs to my room.

I turned off the light and dropped into bed, recklessly stretched and twisted, then curled onto my side as I sunk into about eight inches of memory foam on top of my mattress. After sleeping in so many restricted positions on so many uncomfortable surfaces over the years, I cherished the flexibility that allowed me to be engulfed in the supersoft layer.

Highlighted by the light from the hallway, I could still see the sneakers I'd kicked off just inside my open bedroom door. Seeing those regular shoes and hearing the kids laughing downstairs reminded me of how grateful I was for the ability to be active and for the opportunity to be myself with my family. I had my life back.

I remembered the old Adidas shoes and the devastation they symbolized. The memory of them no longer filled me with panic, as it had for a long time after I stopped wearing them. I knew that I was healed and would never need them again. I was in control of my health.

With a deep sigh of pure joy, I closed my eyes. As I did every night when I went to sleep, I acknowledged a number of things I was thankful for. I was so appreciative not only for my health but also for the knowledge that could help the kids avoid the challenges I'd faced. I was humbled, though, as I recalled a promise I made fifteen years before, when I learned that all cancer had been removed from my body.

I didn't take a minute for granted. I always remembered those who were struggling with something they could not control and from which they may not recover. I knew a little about how it felt to see no way out of an unbearable situation, and was so intensely saddened for people in that position. The perspective I gained was by far the most valuable outcome of my journey.

As I lay in the dark and reflected on my quest to take control of my declining health, I was still shocked that life-changing events could occur through such random, seemingly meaningless acts. Years of tests, diagnoses, and treatments had brought us no closer to understanding my long list of issues.

The simple solution was within my grasp all along. And I found it by accident.

ACKNOWLEDGEMENTS

My health would not be possible without the functional medicine community that taught me so much and helped me reclaim my life. I am forever grateful.

Thanks so much to the talented professionals who helped me put this book together. Nathan Bransford for editing and patiently teaching me how to write, William Drennan for copyediting, and Asya Blue for cover and interior design.

Finally, thanks to my amazing children Gretchen, Kenny, and Chris, for always believing in me.

A NOTE FROM THE AUTHOR

Thank you for reading my story! I wrote *Accidental Health* to provide a different perspective on chronic illness and to raise awareness about the role of food in health. I believe most people have no idea that their very typical lifestyle can make them sick, and never get the information they need to be truly healthy. I hope my book motivates you to learn more, try a healthy change to your diet or lifestyle, find a doctor who is a true partner in your health, or encourage someone you care about to try something different.

Best of luck! It is my sincere wish that something in this book helps you in some way. Let me know. I would love to hear from you!

Dee
www.accidental-health.com
dee@accidental-health.com

Made in the USA
Middletown, DE
27 September 2021

49185174R00125